The Wall Pilates Workout Book For Women

Beautifully Illustrated Step-by-Step Workout Exercises For Toning, Flexibility, Strength, and Balance

Luna Light

The Wall Pilates Workout Book For Women

Beautifully Illustrated Step-by-Step Workout Exercises For Toning, Flexibility, Strength, and Balance

© Copyright 2023 By Luna Light. All rights reserved.

Disclaimer

This book is intended to provide readers with general information about Pilates exercises and routines. The content provided is not a substitute for professional medical advice, diagnosis, or treatment. Engaging in any exercise program carries the risk of injury. While the author and publisher have made every effort to ensure the safety of the exercises and routines described in this book, they cannot guarantee that they are appropriate for every individual. Always seek the advice of a qualified healthcare provider with any questions you may have regarding a medical condition or physical exercise regimen if you are unsure. If you experience pain, dizziness, discomfort, or any other symptoms while performing any of the exercises described in this book, stop immediately and consider seeking medical attention. By voluntarily participating in any of the exercises shown in this publication, you accept the risk of any potential injury. If you are unsure about any exercise, consider seeking advice from a certified Pilates instructor or fitness professional.

Contents

Exercise Group Four

Routines With Control Focus

Exercise Group Five

Pilates Routines With Strength Focus

YOUR BONUS VIDEOS

Congrats! Your new book comes with video lessons included. A lot of time and effort went into making this the best Pilates book and that applies to our videos too. Completed by a certified Pilates instructor, the moves in the videos are correctly done and easy to follow.

Unlike our competitors, you won't have to worry about risking injury, following bad instructions or using improper or dangerous movements.

HOW TO DOWNLOAD YOUR BONUS VIDEOS:
WRITE AN EMAIL TO:
wall.pilates2@gmail.com

Please put in the subject line: **Luna Book 1**

We will unlock and give full access to the video courses shortly once you send that email. Thank you

Your Free Gift

Congrats! Your book comes with 4 bonuses: including the Ultimate Kegels Guide. Just got go wallpilates.org to get them for free.

You may have heard of Kegels before... but unfortunately, there is widespread misinformation about hold time, number of repetitions and how to actually perform the contractions that do more bad than good.

When done right, Kegels are a powerful way to build endurance, increase strength in your core and enhance your sex life. The Kegels exercise we created comes directly from Tim Sawyer, a top physical therapist who worked with doctors at Stanford University[1] to develop rehabilitation programs.

This exact Kegels exercise has helped tremendously in improving my pelvic floor tone, enhancing my sex life, and developing a strong core.

All you have to do is go to wallpilates.org to download it for free. Alternatively, scan the QR code below:

---

1. Dr. Wise and Dr. Anerson authored A Headache in the Pelvis: A New Understanding and Treatment for Chronic Pelvic Pain Syndromes and consulted Tim as the main physical therapist for their treatments.

How You Will Benefit

Practicing Pilates will make you healthier and happier.

Sound too good to be true? Maybe...

But before you start looking for the refund page on Amazon, think about this: millions of people have been doing Pilates since Joseph Pilates' death in 1967, with thousands of different teachers. Some teachers are more memorable and more skilled, others less so. Yet no matter who the teacher is... people continue to learn it. And they stick to it...often for life, more so than any other exercise. Why?

Maybe it's because you feel so good after a workout instead of the "no pain no gain" philosophy of other exercise methods. Maybe it's because once you start learning the movements, you feel taller and more balanced when standing and walking. Maybe people start commenting on how you have good posture and maybe moving around now feels like it just flows instead of being heavy and slow. If you're going through physical therapy or rehabilitation, Pilates is a low risk (less chance of flare-ups or injury) way to improve your strength and posture as you heal.

The Pilates movements in this book ask for your full attention, even when you're performing them alone at home. This level of presence is rare these days in modern society and, in my humble opinion, is desperately needed and surprisingly enjoyable. That's also why I invite you to take a pause whenever you see a lotus symbol, and reflect a moment on what you just read.

With this workbook, all it takes is 15 minutes of exercise per day. Make a promise now to yourself to do at least 10 sessions of your choice of the workout plans included and feel the difference in your body!

Your Friend,
-Luna Light

Origins

"One day everyone in the world will know about Contrology and do it, and we won't need doctors, or hospitals[1]."

— Joseph Pilates

As a child Joseph Pilates was frail and suffered from asthma, rickets, and rheumatic fever. This early life experience fueled his lifelong quest for a holistic approach to health and well-being.

As political tensions rose in Europe, Mr. Pilates emigrated to the United States in the 1920s. Upon arrival in New York City, he and his wife, Clara, opened a fitness studio. This small studio began to attract a diverse clientele, including dancers, actors, and athletes, all drawn to the unique benefits of "Contrology." It was here that his method, later renamed "Pilates" in his honor by his students, began.

After a career spanning over 50 years, on the hospital bed just before his last breath, Mr. Pilates prophesized: "Contrology was perfect, people will awaken to their need of it to survive in the modern world. I was forty years too soon. The world will catch up[2]". Joseph Pilates passed away in 1967, but his legacy lives on in the millions of people today who continue to benefit from the effectiveness of his movements to bring strength and vitality back into their lives.

Today I invite you into the world of Pilates – and to discover this collection of effective and relaxing movements that strengthen, tone, and build flexibility in your body.

---

1. Steel, John Howard. Caged Lion: Joseph Pilates and His Legacy.
2. Steel, John Howard. Caged Lion: Joseph Pilates and His Legacy.

Why Wall Pilates?

"In 10 sessions, you'll feel the difference. In 20, you'll see the difference. And in 30, you'll be on your way to having a whole new body[1]."

— Joseph Pilates

Five years ago, the secrets I learned using Wall Pilates after a car accident helped me get out of chronic pain. At the time I was in so much pain I could not walk and was restricted to my bedroom with a small floor area and wall. Necessity forced me to discover new ways of exercising and getting my life back.

As I recovered from the pain using Pilates movements, I continued to strengthen my body, and I was surprised to find even more health benefits like the ones you'll discover in the following chapter.

Wall Pilates doesn't require complex equipment, is beginner friendly, and space and cost-effective. You can do it anywhere, anytime. Even when I'm traveling without a yoga mat, I simply place a towel on the floor and begin my wonderful workout.

While Yoga and regular Pilates can improve your health, Wall Pilates focuses on using the resistance of the wall to build up your core strength, burn calories, and align and improve your posture. Here's how I explain the difference to prospective students:

Feature	Wall Pilates	Regular Pilates	Yoga
Equipment	Wall, Yoga Mat	Reformer, Wunda Chair, Trapeze Table, Ladder Barrel, and more...	Yoga Mat, Yoga Blocks
Cost	$40 Yoga Mat	$50-100 membership $150 per private session	$40 Yoga Mat
Level Of Difficulty	Beginner To Advanced Beginner Friendly and Senior Friendly	Intermediate to Advanced	Beginner To Advanced
Focus Of Benefits	Core strength, posture, flexibility and pain relief. The wall offers an added dimension of resistance and alignment feedback.	Core strength, coordination, and endurance	Meditation, Flexibility, balance, and mental focus, focusing on inner peace and presence

As you can see, use of the wall grants many advantages. And the good news is… walls are everywhere!

Using the power of the wall, we're able to:

1. **Improve Alignment & Feedback:** The wall provides immediate feedback when you touch it. It can help ensure proper alignment in certain exercises, making it easier to self-identify and correct imbalances or misalignments in the body.
2. **Improve Support**: For some exercises, the wall offers support, making it possible to perform movements that might be challenging on the floor. For example, it can assist in standing leg exercises (example: exercise 30) where balance might be an issue.
3. **Create Resistance**: Pushing or pulling against the wall can add an element of resistance to certain exercises, enhancing their intensity and effectiveness.
4. **Add Variation**: The wall introduces a variety of modifications to traditional Pilates exercises, which can add diversity to a workout routine and target muscles in different ways.

5. **Accessibility**: For those who might find it challenging to get down onto, or up from, the floor or into a machine, the wall provides an accessible alternative.
6. **Space-Efficient**: Using the wall allows people to add variety and challenge to their routines without needing a lot of space or specialized equipment.
7. **Stability and Safety**: For beginners or those recovering from injuries, the wall offers a stable and safe surface to lean on.
8. **Cost Effective**: Instead of paying for expensive equipment and classes, all you need is a yoga mat and a wall.

In essence, the "wall" in Wall Pilates makes it accessible for everyone. That's why so many women, men, seniors, and people recovering from injuries choose this mode of exercise. It's safe, effective, and depending on your situation, sometimes easier to see results compared to traditional methods of working out and rehabilitation:

Why Pilates?	Wall Pilates	Weight Training
Injury Risk	Low impact, less chance of inflammation.	Need resting days, possibility of over-training or straining muscles
Accessibility	People with disabilities, injuries, back pain and pelvic pain can still do Pilates relatively safely with lower risk of "flaring up"	Usually, may need to be younger/healthy to do most intense weight training routines
Intensity	Loving the feeling instead of "forcing it". Less burn out.	Pushing to the limit
Feeling	Connection to breathing, presence and control of whole body	Can feel exhausting or over trained
Diet	Can eat normally and still get results of flexibility, posture, and strength	Some workouts require high caloric intake to build muscle mass
Results	More tonality and strength from the core and body as a holistic, connected unit	Isolates specific muscles. Can become ripped but sometimes at expense of health

This is not to say that weight training can't be performed in combination with Pilates to build muscle, or that one can't transition from one to the other as your goals and life situation changes, but this gives you a good idea of the pros and cons of each exercise method.

With that in mind, I hope you're feeling motivated because next we're going to talk about 7 ways your body will improve in just a few sessions...

---

1. Pilates, Joseph, H.; Miller, William, John. Return to Life Through Contrology.

7 Ways Your Body Will Improve

"Change happens through movement and movement heals."[1]

— Joseph Pilates

1. More Muscle Tone: Pushing or pulling against the wall helps to tone and strengthen various muscle groups, enhancing overall muscle definition. (AKA The "Pilates Body")

2. Better Posture: The wall offers immediate feedback, helping you build spinal awareness and correct postural misalignments. Over time, this can lead to better posture, which is crucial not just for aesthetics but also for reducing strain on the spine and other joints.

3. Improved Flexibility: Leveraging the wall, we can safely deepen the stretches because the wall can support the weight of certain body parts, allowing for extended stretch durations and greater range of motion.

4. Stress Reduction: Pilates emphasizes deep breathing and focused movement. This mindfulness can help alleviate stress as the attention is drawn away from external pressures and directed towards the body's movement and breath. You're so focused you literally don't have time to worry.

5. Sexual Stamina and Flexibility: Improved pelvic floor strength, flexibility, and increased blood flow, all benefits of working your core, can lead to enhanced sexual stamina and flexibility. A strengthened core (that includes the pelvic muscles) can heighten both control and sensation. In fact, Mr. Pilates said in his own words: "So, Contrology strengthens the body and makes it work good for sex. And sex makes people happy and healthier[2]"

6. Improved Mental Acuity: The concentration required in Wall Pilates requires a mindful presence and focus, which helps you improve practice shifting into focus in other areas of your life.

7. Better Sleep: Regular exercise has been linked to improved sleep patterns. Wall Pilates, with its emphasis on relaxation, breathing, and physical exertion, can result in deeper and more restful sleep. You can even use some of the breathing techniques in this book to prime your body for relaxation before going to bed.

Sometimes it's hard for a beginner to see how powerful Pilates movements are, so let's illustrate all the muscles you stimulate in just one movement called "the teaser":

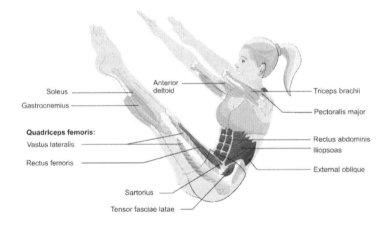

Twelve muscles, type 1 and 2 muscle fibers, small to large.

Remarkable, isn't it?

The concentration, focus and control of these movements will efficiently tone and strengthen multiple muscles in your body.

---

1. Pilates, Joseph, H.; Miller, William, John. Return to Life Through Contrology.
2. Steel, John Howard. Caged Lion: Joseph Pilates and His Legacy.

Avoiding Injuries

"An ounce of prevention is worth a pound of cure."

— Benjamin Franklin

Before we begin, perform a quick check for:

1. A Sturdy Wall: Ensure the wall you're using is solid and can withstand pressure. Avoid walls with loose plaster, as pushing or leaning against them could lead to unexpected breaks or collapses.

2. Clear Space: Ensure the area around the wall is free from obstacles, slippery rugs, glass, or loose items that could lead to trips or falls.

3. Footwear and Attire: Wear appropriate non-slip footwear if you prefer. Pilates is very effective barefoot. Comfortable, form-fitting attire can help you move freely without getting tangled or caught.

4. Staying Hydrated: Drink plenty of water before, during, and after your Wall Pilates session to prevent muscle cramps and promote recovery. I always prepare a water bottle before a workout.

5. Healthy Nutrition: Good nutrition is essential for physical exercises such as Wall Pilates. Your body needs the right nutrients to foster muscle growth and recovery, sustain bone health, and fuel your training sessions. I usually exercise first thing in the morning after hydrating and eat right after.

When exercising, if you feel like you're pushing too hard… it's ok to rest, and then start again, slowly.

Consistency is more important than "going hard."

My mentor once told me: "being extraordinary is simply performing ordinary things consistently over a period of time."

So go at your own pace.

This isn't a race… there's no competition here.

"The focus was all on the doing and not on competing, even with yourself. There were no objective goals such as do more exercises, or faster, or use more resistance. Progress was felt, not measured."

— John Howard Steel: *Caged Lion: Joseph Pilates and His Legacy*

How To Breathe

"Breathing is the first act of life and the last. Our very life depends on it. Since we cannot live without breathing, it is tragically deplorable to contemplate the millions and millions who have never mastered the art of correct breathing."[1]

— Joseph Pilates

There are many nuances to breathwork during Wall Pilates. The most important thing to remember is the <u>coordination of the breath to help the movement of your body.</u> Here are some safe breathing techniques you can experiment with when starting out. Different teachers teach different breathing techniques so try a few and find the one that resonates most with you.

Inhale Through the Nose: Taking a deep breath in, aim to expand the ribcage out to the sides, allowing the lungs to fill up with air.

Exhale Through the Mouth: Purse your lips as if you're blowing out through a straw and exhale fully, engaging your core muscles and feeling the abdominal wall draw inward.

Timing With Movement

As a general rule, exhale during the effort or exertion phase of an exercise and inhale during the return or relaxation phase. For example, when doing a Pilates teaser, you'd exhale as you lift your upper body up toward the sky and inhale as you lower it back down.

Enhancing Stretch and Range

Use your breath to deepen stretches. Typically, inhaling prepares for the movement and exhaling allows you to sink deeper into the stretch.

Using Breath to Expand

Sometimes I go into lightning pose and practice breathing for 10 reps. During each, I imagine my rib cage expanding, then my abdomen, upper back, and lower back. With each breath I see if I can expand my lungs and diaphragm in all directions. After just a few months, this practice has improved my breathing capacity significantly. If you use your mouth to inhale and exhale, you can expand further with more air and then revert back to nose breathing on subsequent counts.

Pacing and Rhythm When Moving

Maintaining a steady breathing rhythm can help set the pace for your exercises. It promotes a mindful approach, preventing rushing through movements and ensuring each exercise is performed with precision.

Cooling Down With 4-7-8 Technique

The 4-7-8 Technique, also known as the "relaxing breath," is a simple breathing exercise developed by Dr. Andrew Weil. It's inspired by an ancient yogic technique called pranayama, which involves the regulation of breath to enhance physical and mental well-being. The 4-7-8 Technique is designed to act as a natural tranquilizer for the nervous system so it's great at the end of a workout. In fact, I use it whenever I feel rushed or stressed outside the gym.

4-7-8 Steps:

1. Inhale quietly through the nose for a count of 4.
2. Hold your breath for a count of 7.
3. Exhale completely through the mouth, making a whoosh sound, for a count of 8.
4. This is 1 breath cycle. Aim to complete this cycle for 4 breaths while you relax.

---

1. Pilates, Joseph, H.; Miller, William, John. Return to Life Through Contrology

How To Feel Good When Moving

"Be fast, but don't hurry."

— John Wooden, legendary UCLA Basketball Coach

Slow movements require more conscious control.

Why? Because slow, controlled movements typically involve more muscle tension over a longer period. This can increase muscle activation, especially in stabilizing muscles, making the exercise more challenging and improving your strength gains.

As you engage with your body in Wall Pilates, you might experience various emotional states. Sometimes, emotions get stuck in our bodies[1]. Embracing these emotions rather than suppressing them can lead to a deeper connection and release.

Wall Pilates cultivates an attitude of patience, kindness, and love toward your body and self, irrespective of your abilities or fitness level. This practice of self-love and acceptance can lead to an improved mental state.

The physical challenge of Wall Pilates can build mental resilience. Each time you overcome a challenging posture or hold a difficult pose for a few breaths longer, you're training your mind to build neuro-connections that you can do it, and that you are stronger than you think.

"Control"

Joseph Pilates called his method "Contrology" A.K.A. "The Art of Control." This is the control of your mind first and then the mind over the body.

I imagine performing the exercises during my walks or even before I do them. As you view the illustrations in this book, imagine watching yourself actually doing them.

After an exercise, try to assess how the movement went. Was it smooth? Could you have held a little longer? Was your posture correct when engaging the movements?

Over time this awareness will get easier and become automatic. You will feel more and more in control and aware of your daily movements and the "humming" of your body and life force.

The "Core"

The "core" is mentioned a lot in Pilates literature. This just means you are moving from your center. Think of the center as this energy field from your abs to your lower back down to your pelvic floor. Every movement in the body involves the ab muscles and the pelvic floor. In fact, the pelvic muscles are the only muscles that never rest except when you're sleeping. By strengthening our center, we're building a solid foundation for freedom in our movements.

I know some of this may sound complicated, but as you make the movements, the truth will come to you.

A great explanation of this "feel-good" movement experience is written by John Howard Steel:

"Pilates is a system of coordinated movement, concentration, and breathing that fully absorbs the actor in what he or she is doing, adds grace and efficiency to daily life, relieves stress, increases circulation, augments self-esteem, becomes a habit, and most importantly is fun to do[2]."

---

1. See "The Body Keeps The Score" by Dr. Van Der Kolk
2. Steel, John Howard. Caged Lion: Joseph Pilates and His Legacy (p. 178). Last Leaf Press. Kindle Edition.

No Equipment? No Problem!

Pilates gyms have a lot of equipment. From resistance bands to foam rollers, to weird names like the "Reformer", "Cadillac" and "Ladder Barrel". Beginners might think we're naming objects in a fantasy game.

These tools and machines can be extremely beneficial in a class setting under a good instructor, however, many of the movements can be carried out at home simply with a wall and yoga mat.

So, let's not get distracted with all the fancy equipment and terminology. In this workout guide, I'm going to help you work out all your core foundational muscles simply using the wall. Of course, a Yoga mat is beneficial to help you gain resistance in certain positions.

This doesn't mean you can't go into a studio and learn how to use (and name) all the amazing equipment that comes in a classic Pilates gym. In fact, at some point you should do so to continue learning and improving.

For now, you can use this workbook to improve your posture, alignment, and strength anywhere you go. Whether you're in your bedroom, staying in a hotel room, even working a late night at the office[1]... all you need is the wall and floor.

Now, let's check out the amazing 28-Day Challenge Workout Plans.

---

1. Just don't put dirty shoes against the office wall and get in trouble with your boss. I have done this myself by taking my shoes off and stretching out during late night work sessions.

The Workout Plans

The following routines refer to each exercise number in this book from 1-56.

Gentle Daily Routine

This is a relaxing routine you can do once a day.

Gentle Daily Routine	Exercise
Warmup	1-6
1	11
2	13
3	15
Rest	7
4	17
5	18
6	19
Rest	8
7	23
8	27
9	28
10	31
Cooldown	10

For Pain Relief

I use this routine every morning when recovering from chronic pain. If you are rehabilitating or recovering from an injury, use this gentle daily routine. Don't be afraid to take a break at any time or even a day off. When starting out… go slow. Because my core was very weak in the beginning, I would perform this routine one day then take the next day off. Eventually, I became strong enough to do this every day.

28-Day Challenge

The following are routines designed to help you achieve a specific goal in 28 days. You can add a rest day after every 3 days of workout for recovery, depending on your fitness level. The rest day does not count towards the "28 Days".

A | Cardio Focus

This challenge focuses on burning calories. Make sure you are eating healthily and staying hydrated. For women, generally the recommended daily calorie intake is 2,000 calories and about 11.5 cups (2.7 liters) of fluids.

Exercise	Day 1-10	Day 11-20	Day 21-28
Warmup	Pick favorite 3	Pick favorite 3	Pick favorite 3
1	11	22	13
2	12	21	14
3	14	20	17
Resting pose	8	7	8
4	13	19	21
5	16	18	22
6	18	17	18
Resting pose	10	8	7
7	17	23	46
8	19	24	48
9	21	40	51
10	20	41	54
Cooldown	9	9	9

B | Control Focus

This challenge is great for improving flexibility and posture.

Exercise	Day 1-10	Day 11-20	Day 21-28
Warmup	Pick favorite 3	Pick favorite 3	Pick favorite 3
1	23	36	32
2	24	25	25
3	26	38	31
Resting pose	7	7	7
4	27	34	33
5	28	35	35
6	29	39	36
Resting pose	8	8	8
7	30	40	44
8	31	41	45
9	32	42	51
10	33	43	57
Cooldown	9	9	9

C | Strength Focus

This challenge builds strength while increasing flexibility and posture. Exercises 50 and 56 require a higher level of skill with handstands so please seek a professional instructor if you're new.

Exercise	Day 1-10	Day 11-20	Day 21-28
Warmup	Pick favorite 3	Pick favorite 3	Pick favorite 3
1	21	51	54
2	22	52	52
3	23	53	51
Resting pose	9	9	9
4	24	54	53
5	26	56	55
6	27	57	56
Resting pose	8	8	8
7	44	24	50
8	45	25	49
9	48	26	48
10	51	54	54
Cooldown	7	7	7

For strength training, whenever your muscles become really sore, take a day off, even two if needed for recovery. I started out performing two days of training and taking one day off. Listen to your body and go at your own pace. Remember this is not a race.

My Chronic Pain Story

Years ago, a car accident sent me to the ER at UCLA with a stabbing-like pain in my abdominal wall and pelvic floor. The doctors could not find anything wrong but what followed was months of tests, MRIs, blood draws, and hospital visits. Even with all that, no one could tell me what was wrong with my body or why I was in pain. I spent the next two years searching for a way to cure my chronic pain syndrome[1].

While many things contributed to my healing, when I began doing Pilates... I immediately started feeling better. After my first few sessions, the changes I experienced in my body made me realize that there was a way to fully recover.

While everyone's body's different, and chronic pain can have overlapping and complicated causes, I discovered my chronic pain was coming from weak muscles riddled with Trigger Points (TrPs). These are taut muscle bands that restrict movement and blood flow. If you feel like you have Trigger Points, a great place to start is Claire Davis's book **The Trigger Point Therapy Workbook**.

So, if you have muscles ridden with Trigger Points like I did, you must first get rid of those TrPs. But what comes later is a weak, TrPs free muscle. This is where Pilates comes in. The ability of Pilates to exercise all the slow and fast twitch muscle fibers, and to control smaller muscles that regular exercises don't stimulate to the same level, is how I trained my weak muscles to become stronger.

As I improved my precision in my Pilates exercises, the pelvic and abdominal pain slowly faded away. The origin of the pain and dysfunction – weak and TrP-ridden muscles, started to disappear.

I'm now pain-free thanks to Pilates, and it continues to improve my strength, stamina, sex life, and mental well-being. I hope it can do the same for you.

---

1. Pain becomes "chronic" when it lasts more than 6 months without a proper diagnosis.

Before We Begin, 4 Tips:

Slow Down

In Pilates, we slow down to get results faster. Slow, controlled movements typically involve more muscle strength, control, and posture gains.

Focus

Concentrate your attention on the whole movement.

Breathe

Let your breath synchronize with your movement, like a dance.

Relax

Need a break? You can rest anytime by going into one of the resting positions.

Exercise Group One
Warmup Routines

A proper warmup gently activates your muscles. It gets the blood flowing and improves joint lubrication. All of this prevents potential injuries.

I know most people skip warmups.

I don't blame you. When I first started, I thought warmups were for "weak people" and that I would just "skip to the good part."

Later I learned (the hard way) … skipping warmups is a recipe for getting injured.

Instead, think of warmups as a fun game.

During warmup, we are gifted the opportunity to get mentally ready, and bring conscious awareness to the control of your breath and your body.

So, every time you start a workout session, begin with 3 of your favorite warmups from this section. You can even perform all 6 of them. They are easy and feel great.

1 | Wall Cow Pose

The cow pose can be modified using the wall as resistance pushing against the feet for an optimal stretch of your entire upper body.

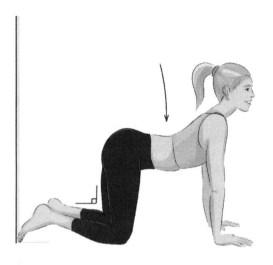

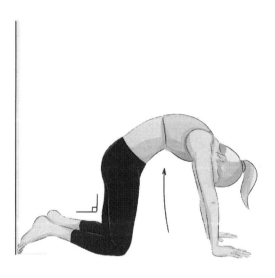

Wall Cow Pose Instructions

Starting Position

Begin on all fours in a tabletop position on your mat. Push your toes against the wall for additional resistance and stability. Ensure your wrists are aligned directly under your shoulders and your knees under your hips.

Note: the wall is optional only if you need more stability.

Pose 1

As you inhale, arch your spine by dropping your belly towards the mat. Lift your head and tailbone towards the ceiling, creating a gentle curve in your back. Ensure you are not straining your neck. The movement should feel natural.

Pose 2

As you exhale, arch your spine and drop your head. Relax here for 3 seconds.

Repeat both poses for 5 relaxing reps.

Tips:

- If you are recovering from back pain, start very slowly and only go as far as comfortable.
- Be careful not to throw out your neck by looking upward. Imagine your neck and spine as one holistic unit working together.

2 | Wall Leg Stretch

The wall leg stretch is a fantastic exercise to lengthen and stretch the hamstrings, calves, and lower back.

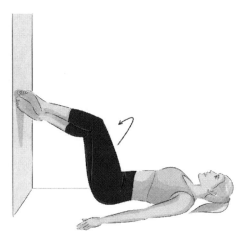

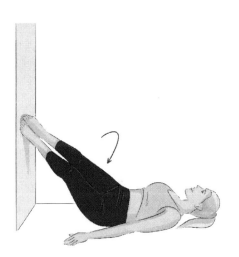

Wall Leg Stretch Instructions

Starting Position

Lie on your back on a comfortable surface or mat, placing your feet securely against the wall at a 45-degree angle.

Pose 1

As you inhale, use your toes to guide you and turn to the right with both legs. Exhale freely and maintain the position for 5 seconds.

Pose 2

Release to starting position. Now repeat the same movement on the left side with both legs. Maintain for 5 seconds.

Repeat the left and right movement 5 times on each side for ten total movements. Only go as far as you comfortably can. If this feels relaxing, sometimes I continue this until my whole lower body feels loose and relaxed.

Tips:

- If you have back or pelvic pain, be careful not to overextend on this exercise. Turn only left or right to a comfortable range for you.
- Keep your head against the floor when you do this. Make sure your spine is aligned and the weight is fully dropped, like you're melting into the floor.

3 | Wall Staff Pose

This exercise stretches your back and aligns your shoulder and lower back for better posture. It can also be used as a great resting position after a workout.

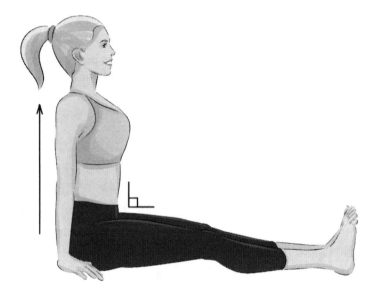

Wall Staff Pose Instructions

Starting Position

Lean your head and butt firmly against the wall. Place your hands to the side with fingers pointing forward and toes up.

Pose 1

Extend your spine. Imagine you are becoming as tall as possible, without forcing it.

Stay here for up to 30 seconds.

Tips:

- Remember to keep your toes pointed up.
- A variation of this is to place your hands on your lap. You may recognize this pose in the Egoscue Method. Make sure your shoulders are aligned between the left and right and maintain contact with the wall throughout.

4 | Scapula Stretch

The scapula, commonly known as the shoulder blade, plays a pivotal role in the functioning of the shoulder and upper back. Stretching the muscles attached to and surrounding the scapula increases muscular balance in the upper body and improves posture and mobility.

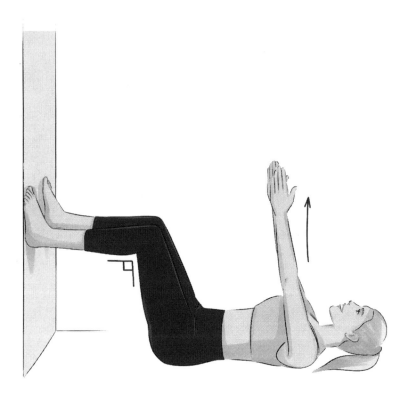

Scapula Stretch Instructions

Starting Position

Lie on your back with your foot resting firmly against the wall at a 90-degree angle. Raise your arms straight up, head laying softly against the floor/mat.

Pose 1

As you inhale, extend the hands upward and hold for 2 seconds.

Pose 2

As you exhale, release, and move your hand back to the original position. Repeat for 10 reps.

Tips:

- Let your hands guide you. As you move the hands, the shoulder follows by natural extension.
- Keep your head against the floor. Remember this is not a sit up. We are isolating the arm and shoulders.

5 | Wall Arm Windmill

This is a beautiful stretch of your entire arm that relaxes your shoulders down to the hands.

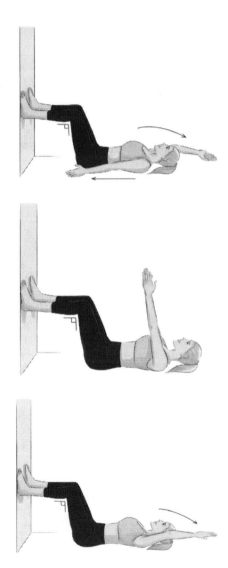

Wall Arm Windmill Instructions

Starting Position

Lie on your back with your foot resting firmly against the wall at a 45-degree angle. Raise 1 arm upward on the floor and place the other firmly towards the wall.

Pose 1

As you inhale, move both arms towards the center simultaneously.

Pose 2

As you exhale, release, and move your arms back to the floor, reversing the original arm positions.

Repeat this movement for a total of 10 reps.

Tips:

- Use your breath for guidance and remember to keep your head firmly on the floor.

6 | Wall Leg Stretch

The wall leg stretch focuses on the hamstrings, calves, and the muscles in the lower back.

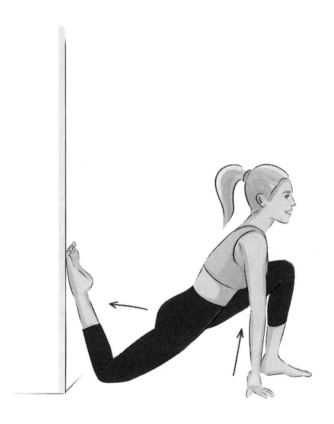

Wall Leg Stretch Instructions

Starting Position

Put your right foot against the wall and your left leg bent while lunging forward.

Place your right arm on the floor for balance.

Head looking forward. Hold for 30 seconds.

During this time use your breath to see if you can extend further forward.

Switch Sides

Change sides. If you started with your right foot and right arm, now change to the left foot against the wall and left hand on the floor.

Hold for 30 seconds.

Tips:

- Keep your hands on the floor for stability and your head looking forward.
- Experiment with how far away from the wall you can be. The optimal distance offers a great stretch in your quad muscles.

Exercise Group Two
Resting Positions

Resting positions give your body a chance to relax and recover.

They can be performed after every 3-5 exercises, or whenever you feel like you need to rest.

Never be afraid to stop and go into a resting position.

Listen to your body and become present with it.

Remember that in Pilates it's not about "going all out." We're seeking the perfect balance of movement, awareness, and concentration.

7 | Happy Baby

A gentle hip opener and a back stretch that can be both relaxing and rejuvenating.

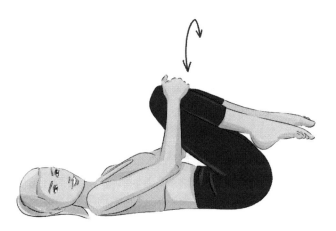

Happy Baby Instructions

Knees to Chest: Lying on the floor, bend your knees and bring them towards your chest.

Hold Your Feet: Reach up to grab the outer edges of your knees with your hands.

Gentle Rock: If it feels good, you can gently rock from side to side, or up and down, massaging your back against the floor.

Hold and Release: Stay in this pose for anywhere from 30 seconds to a few minutes, depending on your comfort. To come out of the pose, gently release your feet and lay them down on the mat.

Tips:

- Once you're in the pose, take deep breaths, and relax. Let gravity help deepen the hip opening, but don't force anything.
- I like to start out rocking side to side until I can learn to maintain my balance, then I rock front to back.

8 | Child's Pose

A restorative yoga posture that promotes relaxation and stretches the back.

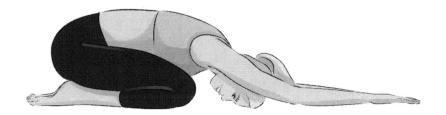

Child's Pose Instructions

Start on All Fours: Begin in a tabletop position with your wrists under your shoulders and your knees under your hips.

Sit Back: Push your hips back toward your heels, lowering your torso between your thighs.

Extend Arms: Stretch your arms out in front, palms facing down on the floor.

Rest Your Forehead: Bring your forehead to the ground.

Relax: Breathe deeply and relax in this position, allowing your back to stretch and your mind to calm.

Hold: Stay in this pose for up to a minute.

Sometimes I stay here for a few minutes because it feels so wonderful!

9 | Corpse Pose

A deep relaxation pose that's ideal for cooling down after a workout and enabling total muscle relaxation.

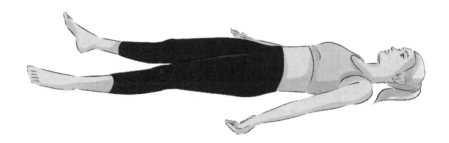

Corpse Pose Instructions

Start Lying Down: Begin by lying flat on your back on a yoga mat or a soft surface.

Legs Apart: Let your feet fall open naturally, positioning them approximately hip-width apart or wider.

Arms at Sides: Place your arms alongside your body, but slightly apart from it. Palms face upwards, allowing the fingers to curl naturally.

Relax Your Body: Release any tension from the body. Let your muscles soften and melt into the floor. The weight of your body is no longer yours – let the floor carry the burden.

Stay in this position for up to 60 seconds. If doing this after a full workout routine, you can stay here for up to 5 minutes.

Tips:

- Neutral Neck: Ensure your neck is in a neutral position. If necessary, place a small pillow or rolled towel under your head to support the natural curve of your neck.
- Breathe Naturally: Focus on your breathing. Allow it to be natural and effortless. Notice the rise and fall of your chest and abdomen.

10 | Thunderbolt Pose

A kneeling pose often used for meditation and to catch your breath. Excellent if you are practicing breathing exercises.

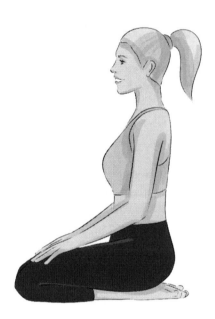

Thunderbolt Pose Instructions

Start by kneeling on the floor or a yoga mat. Keep your feet together with the big toes touching.

Sit Back: Sit back so that your buttocks are resting on your heels. The tops of your feet should be flat on the floor.

Spine Straight: Ensure that your spine is straight and erect. Imagine a line of energy traveling up your spine, through the crown of your head.

Hands on Thighs: Place your hands on your thighs, palms facing down.

Relax Shoulders: Drop your shoulders down and away from your ears and relax them.

Head and Neck: Keep your head straight, with your gaze directed forward. If you're using the pose for meditation, you can close your eyes.

Tips:

- This pose is often cited in Yoga practices to help digestion by promoting proper gastrointestinal function.
- Often used as a base pose ensuring an erect spine.
- Strengthens the back and legs.

Exercise Group Three
Routines With Cardio Focus

There are many benefits of cardiovascular exercise from improved metabolism, improved lung capacity, and improved sleep... the list goes on.

If you've heard the term "Pilates Body," it's because the following exercises not only use cardio to burn calories but they also strengthen and tone your muscle groups at the same time.

That said...it's important to remember that Pilates is a system developed by Joseph Pilates that involves low-impact exercises designed to strengthen muscles, improve postural alignment, and enhance flexibility. So, while not specifically designed for weight loss, it's a very visible secondary effect.

Best of all, you'll feel stronger, more flexible, and move with more aligned posture.

11 |Wall Leg Raise To Back Kick

This routine activates your glutes, lower back and strengthens your leg muscles.

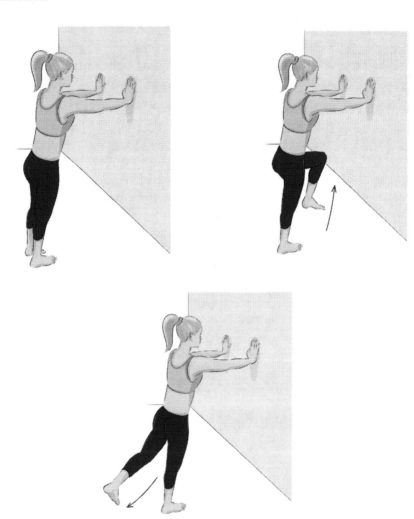

Wall Leg Raise To Back Kick Instructions

Start Position

Stand upright next to a wall and place both hands on the wall for balance. Stand close enough to easily touch the wall without leaning into it.

Pose 1

Slowly lift your left leg as high as you can. Hold this position for 2 seconds.

Pose 2

With a controlled movement, now move your left leg backward, almost like a slow kick away from the wall. Engage your glute muscles and thighs and go as far as you can. Hold here for 2 seconds.

Repeat this 5 times then switch to the right leg and repeat again for a total of 10 reps.

Tips:

- Use controlled movements rather than relying on momentum.

12 | Wall Marches

Wall Marches in Pilates focuses on control, stability, and awareness rather than intensity or speed. Ensure you maintain proper alignment and engagement throughout the exercise.

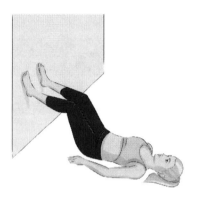

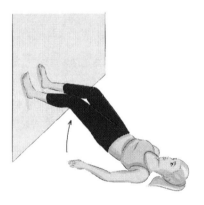

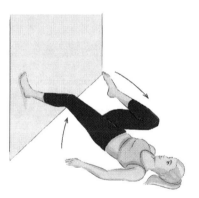

Wall Marches Instructions

Starting Position

Place both feet against the wall while lying flat.

Pose 1

Push off the wall until your butt is pointing upward. Place your arms on the ground to stabilize your arched back.

Pose 2

Slowly lift your right leg towards your chest as far as comfortable. Ensure your pelvis remains stable and doesn't tilt or rotate.

Lower the right foot back to the wall.

Repeat

Repeat the same movement with your left leg.

Aim for 8-10 lifts with each leg, maintaining pelvic stability throughout the exercise.

Tips:

- Focus on keeping the pelvis steady. Imagine if you had to balance a glass of water on your pelvis.
- The wall provides tactile feedback, helping you become aware of any unnecessary movements or shifts in the spine or pelvis.
- Ensure that the movement comes from the hip joint and not by arching the lower back.

13 | Wall Plank

The wall plank is more beginner friendly than a regular plank, while still improving your upper body strength and flexibility.

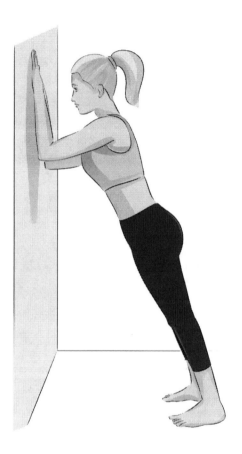

Wall Plank Instructions

Starting Position

Place your hands and forearms flat against the wall, slightly wider than shoulder-width apart.

Lean In: Walk your feet back and then lean into the wall.

Your body should be at an incline, with your weight supported by your hands and forearms. Ensure your body forms a straight line from your head to your heels.

Hold: Maintain this plank position. Keep your core engaged.

Breathe: Breathe steadily. Avoid holding your breath.

Duration: To begin, aim to hold the plank for 20-30 seconds, gradually increasing in duration as you become stronger.

Return: To come out of the plank, walk your feet towards the wall and stand upright.

Tips:

- Avoid sagging in the lower back or hiking the hips up. Maintain a straight line.
- Keep your head in a neutral position, in line with the spine.

14 | Wall Push Up

Wall push-ups are a fantastic modification of the traditional push-up, making it accessible for beginners, those with limited upper body strength, or individuals rehabilitating from injuries.

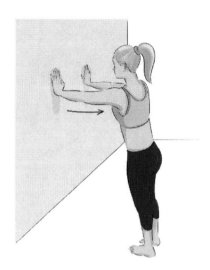

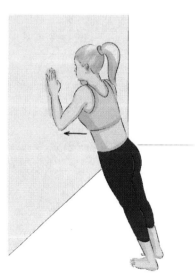

Wall Push Up Instructions

Starting Position

Stand facing a wall with your feet hip-width apart and about 1.5 to 2 feet away, depending on your height. Place your hands flat on the wall, slightly wider than shoulder-width apart. Your hands should be at chest height or slightly below, with fingers pointing upward.

Inhale to Prepare: Take a deep breath in preparation.

Exhale and Bend: As you exhale, bend your elbows, and lean your body toward the wall, keeping your feet on the ground.

Inhale to Push Away: Now press your hands into the wall, straightening your elbows and returning to the starting position as you inhale.

Repetitions: Perform the exercise for 8-12 repetitions depending on strength level.

Tips:

- As you bend your elbows, ensure they don't flare out too widely.
- As you become stronger and more confident, you can challenge yourself by standing farther from the wall and holding the bend position for longer before pushing away. (I started with 1 second, then held for 2 seconds, and now I can hold for 3 seconds each time I learn inward for 10 reps.)

15 | Wall Calf Raises

This is a great exercise for posture alignment and strengthening the calf muscles.

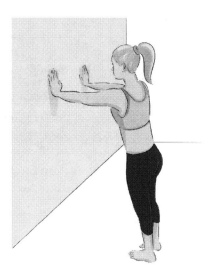

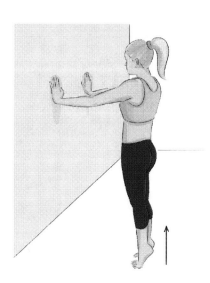

Wall Calf Raises Instructions

Starting position

Stand facing a wall with feet hip-width apart and arms comfortably extended against the wall.

Pose 1

Place hands on the wall for balance. As you inhale, rise onto the balls of your feet, lifting heels as high as possible. Hold for 2 seconds.

Pose 2

On the exhale, slowly lower heels back to the ground.

Repeat for 10 repetitions.

Variation

You can isolate each leg and raise only 1 at a time. Be sure to repeat the same number of lifts for the other calf.

Tips:

- The initial pose uses the wall to remind your body of a straight spine.

16 | Wall Lateral Lunge

Using a wall for guidance and support, this routine can help strengthen your glutes, adductors, and legs.

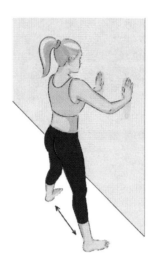

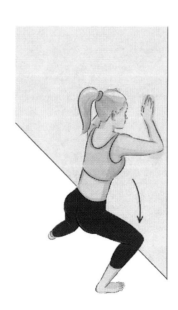

Wall Lateral Lunge Instructions

Starting Position

Place your hands on the wall and feet wide apart.

Pose 1

With a controlled movement, bend your right leg and go as far as comfortable. As you move use your hands to guide your whole body to the right. Try to keep your left leg straight as possible.

Pose 2

Move back to the center and repeat the lunge with the left leg. Repeat 5 times on each leg for a total of 10 reps.

Tips:

- Depth: Go as deep into the lunge as your flexibility and strength allow while keeping good form. Over time, as your flexibility and strength improve, you'll be able to sink deeper into the lunge.
- Foot Stability: Ensure the foot of your lunging leg remains flat on the ground throughout the movement. Avoid lifting the heel or rolling to the outer edge of the foot.

17 | Wall Twist

A beautiful upper body stretch that loosens the spine, shoulders, and arms.

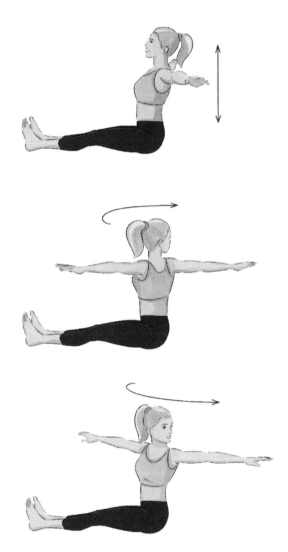

Wall Twist Instructions

Starting Position

Sit with your legs straight and together on the ground. Feet touching or slightly apart is fine. The wall is optional, but you can put both feet against it for balance. Extend arms out at shoulder height.

Note: the wall is optional if you need help keeping your legs in place and lowered to the floor.

Pose 1

Inhale and turn the body to the right and extend as far as comfortable.

Pose 2

Exhale and rotate now to center and then turn the body to the left and extend as far as comfortable.

Repeat turns 8times for a thorough stretch of the arms and upper body.

If you're having trouble keeping your legs straight, it's ok to bend them a little bit.

Tips:

- Keep Hips Stable: Your hips should remain square and facing forward throughout the movement. The twist should come from the thoracic (upper) spine and not the lumbar (lower) spine.
- Stay Upright: Ensure you remain tall and avoid leaning forward or backward during the twist.

18 | Straight Legged Sit Ups

A simple and effective core strengthening exercise.

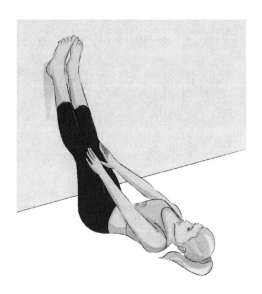

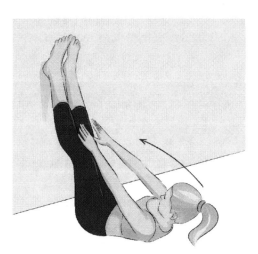

Straight Legged Sit Ups Instructions

Starting position

Lie on your back with legs straight up against the wall and feet together. Place hands on your knees.

Pose 1

Engage core and lift your head off the ground, keeping legs stationary.

Move your hands upward as far as you can comfortably, moving from your core.

Pose 2

Slowly lower back down to the starting position.

Repeat for 10 repetitions. You can inhale when lowering down and exhale when going upward.

Tips:

- When starting out focus on performing each repetition with good form rather than trying to carry out as many as possible. Quality reps will be more effective in targeting the right muscles.

19 | Wall Leg Swings

Leg swings are an excellent way to increase hip and leg flexibility and mobility.

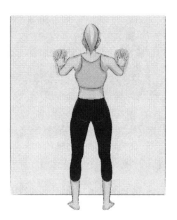

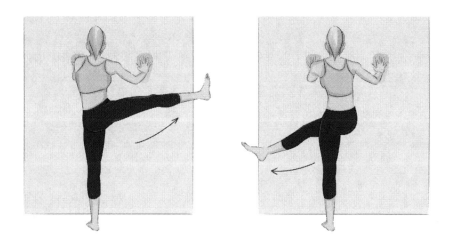

Wall Leg Swings Instructions

Starting position

Stand straight facing the wall and extend your arms so they push against it. Make sure there is enough space for your legs to swing between you and the wall.

Pose 1

Extend your right leg as far upward to the right as possible while maintaining balance.

Pose 2

Slowly rotate your right leg clockwise and now swing left. Go as far as you comfortably can.

Repeat pose 1 and 2 for 10 full swings.

Repeat with the left leg for ten swings for a total of 20 reps.

Tips:

- Start with small swings and build up to longer swings to get accustomed to the exercise.
- You can contract your abdominal muscles to maintain a straight back.

20 | Wall Angels

A popular exercise often prescribed by physical therapists and fitness professionals to address postural issues, particularly for individuals who spend extended periods sitting or working at a desk.

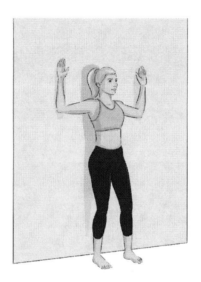

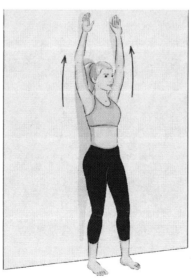

Wall Angels Instructions

Starting Position

Begin by standing with your entire back pressed against a wall. Your feet should be about hip-width apart and positioned a few inches away. This stance helps maintain a neutral spine.

Pose 1

Hold your arms up with a 90-degree angle at your elbows. Use the wall for guidance and resistance support.

Pose 2

Extend your arms upward. Drop back down to pose 1.

A variation is to extend upward and then bring your hands together in a prayer pose pointing to the sky. Then drop back down to pose 1.

Repeat for 10 reps.

Tips:

- If you're having trouble or rehabilitating from an injury, prioritize form over range of motion. As your shoulder mobility improves, the movement may become easier.
- As you gain strength and postural awareness you can do this without wall support.

21 | Wall Teaser

Using the wall, we can add support while improving strength, balance, and coordination of the core muscles.

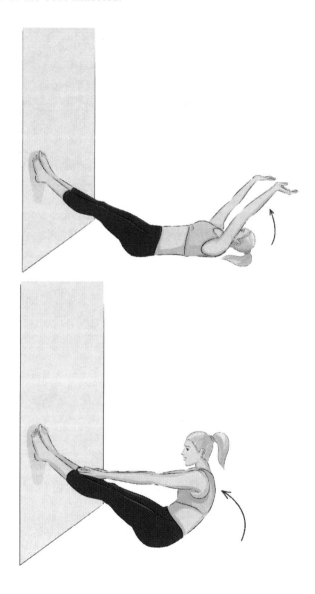

Wall Teaser Instructions

Starting Position

Begin by laying down, feet facing the wall.

Pose 1

Place your feet up against the wall.

Pose 2

Start by raising your arms over your head. Next, engage your core muscles and move your arms towards the wall.

As your hands move above your head, engage your core, and raise your head like you are doing a sit up until facing the wall.

Reach your hands as far as you can up towards your feet. You don't have to touch your legs or your feet, just feel the core movement upward and toward the wall.

Return

When finished, return your spine to the floor as you slowly reverse the action by lowering your head and arms to the starting position (arms still in the air above head).

Repeat for 10 reps.

Tips:

- If you find it difficult to keep your legs straight, you can bend your knees slightly to help with the movement.

22 | Wall Assisted Half Body Plank

This plank variation uses the wall and your arms for additional stability.

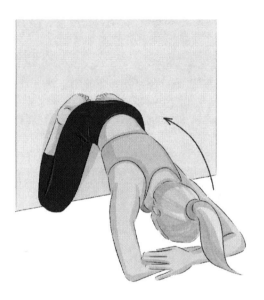

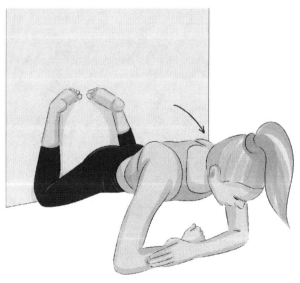

Wall Assisted Half Body Plank Instructions

Starting Position

Start in a kneeling position on a mat. Move back and extend your legs up the wall, bending them while extending into a downward dog with your head down and arms as a resting point against the floor.

Pose 1

Slowly move forward into a plank position. Keep your head relaxed and look towards the ground.

Repeat for 8-10 reps.

Tips:

- Inhale on the return and exhale when extending out for breath control.
- Maintain Neck Position: Ensure that your neck remains neutral and aligned with your spine. Avoid craning your neck upwards or letting it droop downwards.
- Shoulder Stability: Engage the muscles around your shoulder blades (scapula) to ensure stability and prevent sagging.
- Avoid Arching the Lower Back: The activation of your core muscles should prevent the lower back from arching. Ensure your lower back remains neutral throughout the exercise.

Exercise Group Four
Routines With Control Focus

Joseph Pilates chose the name "Contrology" because he believed his system used the mind to control the body. In this context, "control" means the conscious, deliberate movement and command over one's body.

That's why the exercises in Pilates, or Contrology, are not about doing rapid, high-repetition sets, but rather about performing slower, precise movements with full muscular control.

In fact, some Pilates instructors ban use of the word "exercise" and instead use the word "movement" in their books and trainings (you may have noticed that little pattern reading this book).

In either case, we know that this level of control works fast-twitch muscle fibers (type-2) and slow-twitch muscle fibers (type-1) and reduces the risk of injury while giving you tone, strength and flexibility that other movements cannot.

This section includes exercises that improves your control focus of the movements.

23 | The Wall Roll Up

A beautiful exercise that practices slow and deliberate control of the upper body. Great for your spine.

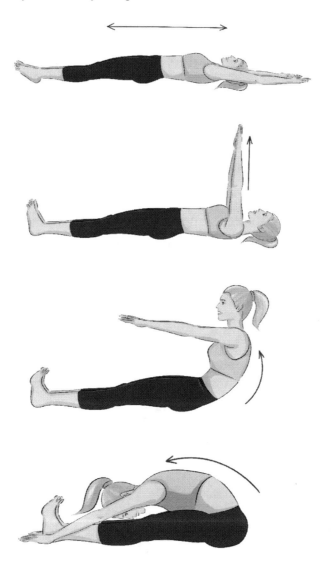

The Wall Roll Up Instructions

Starting Position

Lie flat and let the weight of your entire body rest on the floor. Stretch your arms straight backward and place your toes against the wall.

The wall is optional in this pose, use it to help gain resistance to help with this movement and to keep your legs straight. As you gain flexibility remove the wall and stretch your hands out further than your toes in the last movement.

Pose 1

As you inhale, bring arms straight up with toes pointing upward.

Pose 2

As you exhale slowly, bring your chin down and head forward.

Pose 3

While exhaling slowly, roll forward as much as you comfortably can and hold for 10 seconds. You can do a back-and-forth rock here with the stretch and see if you can reach just a little further each time.

Repeat the poses 4 times and remember to breathe slowly while moving. Use the breath to guide you through the movements. See if you can go further each time.

Tips:

- When lying down (pose 1), your entire spine must touch the mat and make sure you are fully extended and not tense.
- As you come up, press both legs and try to keep them against floor. If you can't, don't sweat the small stuff. Lift them slightly and keep practicing until you can keep both legs against the floor.
- Don't worry if you can't extend all the way down with your head and hands, just stretch as far as you can.

24 | The Spine Stretch

This beautiful pose stretches your entire spine.

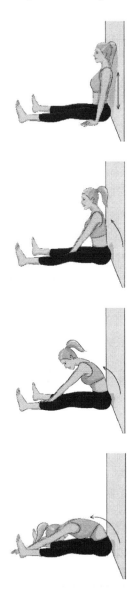

The Spine Stretch Instructions

Starting Position

Spread legs apart as wide as possible while placing your back straight against the wall. Toes pointed upward, rest your palms on each side of the floor.

Pose 1

Begin stretching forward with each "slide" moving forward a little bit until you can reach as far as possible.

Pose 2

When you reach your limit, try extending your arms as far as you comfortably can and hold for 8 seconds.

Repeat for 3 repetitions and try to see if you can go a little further each time.

Tips:

- The initial pose uses the wall to remind your body of a straight spine. Starting from a relaxed, straight posture ensures the rest of the exercise goes correctly.
- Keep your head and neck relaxed while extending forward. If you tense the neck and head, it adds more pressure. The whole body, from head to pelvic floor, should feel like a slow, relaxed stretch.
- Take slow, controlled deep breaths as needed. You can breathe in and out of your mouth for more power to expand and extend your chest area, which will also help your flexibility over time.
- Don't worry if your flexibility is limited when starting out. Stretch as far as you comfortably can.

25 | The Control Balance

This exercise improves your balance and gives an amazing stretch to your legs and core.

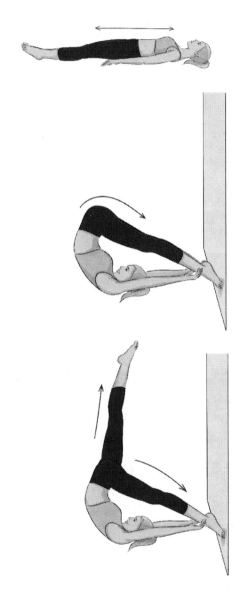

The Control Balance Instructions

Starting Position

Begin lying on your back with feet pointing away from the wall.

Pose 1

Now raise your legs and bring them in over your head and hold your feet (or ankles) firmly with your hands. Use the wall for balance if needed.

Pose 2

Now lift 1 leg straight up (e.g., left leg) to the ceiling while using your hands to keep hold of the other leg (e.g., right leg). Go slowly, feeling the movement of every muscle. If you can't fully extend your leg, it's ok to bend it a bit.

The wall can be used as a backstop if you're having issues with balance but it's optional.

Pose 3

Now bring the upward facing leg back (e.g., left leg) and switch leg positions. At any point, use the wall if you need to rest or fall out of balance.

Repeat this for both legs 3 times each (6 total).

Tips:

- If you can't keep your legs straight, don't worry. Bend them a bit and just go through this movement slowly.
- The wall will assist you as a beginner and be a safety net if you lose balance... but don't overdo it. As you get better you can move further from the wall and only use it if your legs get tired or lose balance.
- If you're unsure when first attempting, consider guidance from a certified Pilates instructor.

26 | Kneeling Chest Raise

This exercise targets the muscles in the chest, shoulders, and core.

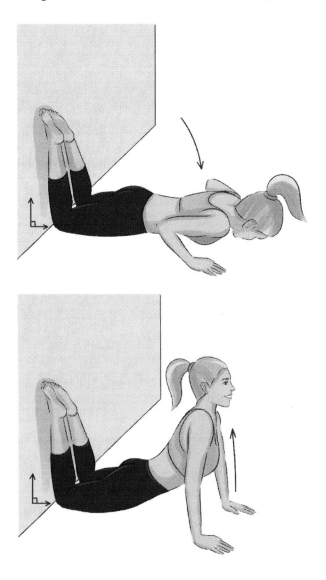

Kneeling Chest Raise Instructions

Starting Position

Begin lying down with your lower legs pressed against the wall, head facing downward.

Pose 1

Slowly push upward and raise your chest. Keep your head gaze facing forward.

Hold for 5 seconds and then return to starting position.

Repeat for 8 reps.

This is like the cobra pose but with legs pressed against the wall.

Tips:

- Maintain core engagement so you don't hyperextend the back.
- Move within a range comfortable for you.

27 | Wall Downward Dog

Instead of placing hands and feet on the ground, in this modification the wall adds support against the feet making the pose more accessible to beginners or those with limitations.

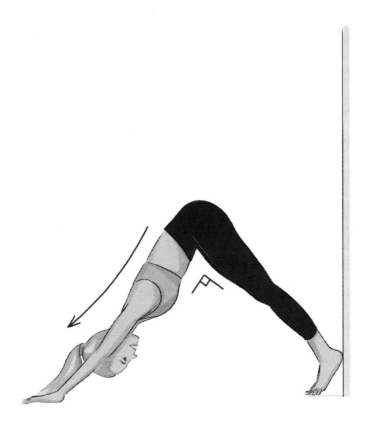

Wall Downward Dog Instructions

Starting Position

Start with your back against the wall and lean forward, touching the ground with your hands.

Pose 1

Move your hands slowly forward using the wall as support against your feet. Move as far as you comfortably can.

Pose 2

Now extend your back upwards and backwards as far as you comfortably can, keeping your head loose in a straight line down the spine.

Press into the floor with your chest and up into the air with your buttocks. Hold and breathe for 15 seconds.

Tips:

- I inhale as I move forward and exhale as I press into my feet.
- The distance between your hip bones and your head determines the length of the stretch. On each breath, see if you can go just a little further.

28 | High Lunge Pose

A lovely stretch for the neck and upper body that helps you find balance in the lower body.

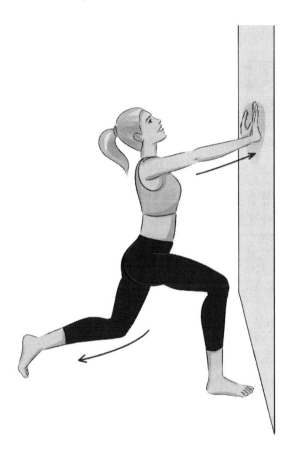

High Lunge Pose Instructions

Starting Position

Start in a standing position facing the wall.

Pose 1

Step one foot back as far as you can with heel slightly lifted. Bend the knee slightly on the other leg. Place your hands against the wall.

Pose 2

Extend and move your head upward and extend your neck upward and backward. Stay comfortable and do this slowly. Hold here for 3 breaths.

Pose 3

Reverse leg positions and repeat 3 times for a total of 6 reps between both legs.

To Release

Exit the pose by lowering your arms and stepping your extended foot forward, returning to a standing position.

Tips:

- Stay in the High Lunge Pose for at least 3 breaths, ensuring your spine remains long, core engaged, and hips square to the front of your mat.

29 | Wall Side Plank

A safe and easy way to stretch your core and sides.

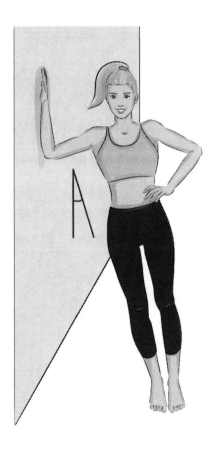

Wall Side Plank Instructions

Starting Position

Stand sideways about an arm's length from a wall. Extend the arm closest to the wall and place your hand on the wall at a comfortable height. Place the other hand on your waist.

Pose 1

Stack your feet together and shift weight onto the foot closest to the wall. Hold for 10 seconds.

Pose 2

Switch sides and hold for 10 seconds, repeating for both sides twice each.

Tips:

- As you hold the pose, work on expanding breaths.
- Adjust Hand Height: If you have shoulder discomfort, you can adjust your hand's height on the wall to find a more comfortable position.
- Adjust Distance From Wall: You can reduce the distance from the wall for easier movement and extend further out the better you become.

30 | Supported Warrior 3

A fantastic pose for improving balance, strengthening the standing leg, and toning the muscles of the lifted leg.

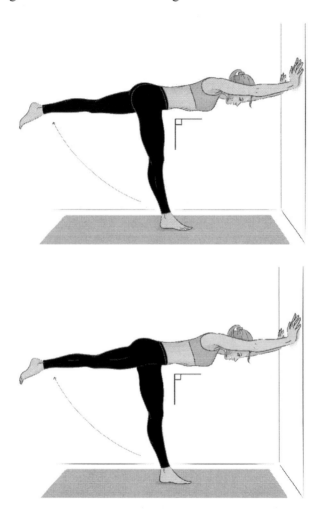

Supported Warrior 3 Instructions

Starting Position

Bend over facing the wall and place your hands on wall with your arms straight.

Pose 1

Shift weight to one foot (e.g., left).

Slowly lift the other leg (e.g., right), keeping a straight back and hips square.

Tilt your upper body forward toward the ground until you can maintain a straight line from head to lifted heel (180 degrees).

Pose 2

Hold for several breaths. I take 5 deep inhales and exhales.

Slowly return to standing by lowering the leg that's raised.

Repeat for the opposite side.

Tips:

- Steady Breathing: Maintaining a consistent breathing pattern can help with balance and focus.
- Flexibility in Support: If using a wall feels too easy, you can transition to using just 1 hand for support or try the pose without any support as you become more comfortable.

31 | Wall Downard Facing Dog

This variation offers many of the same benefits as the traditional pose but with a different level of intensity and control for the smaller back muscles.

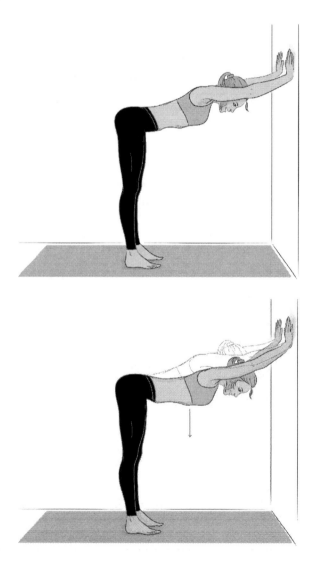

Wall Downard Facing Dog Instructions

Starting Position

Stand facing a wall, about an arm's length away. Comfortably place hands on wall above your head. Slowly slide down with your arms and bow your head to the wall.

Pose 1

Press chest towards the ground, keeping ears aligned with upper arms. Push hips back, legs straight, and heels grounded.

Pose 2

Engage core and hold for 3 deep breaths. Return to standing to release.

Repeat 3 times.

Tips:

- Avoid Hyperextension: Be mindful not to lock your elbows or knees. A tiny, soft bend can prevent hyperextension.
- Adjust Distance for Comfort: Depending on your height and flexibility, you may need to adjust how far you stand from the wall or how high your hands are placed.
- Flexibility Considerations: If you're more flexible, you might find that placing your hands lower on the wall (closer to waist height) offers a deeper stretch.

32 | Puppy Dog Wall Pose

A heart-opening stretch that primarily targets the spine, shoulders, and upper body.

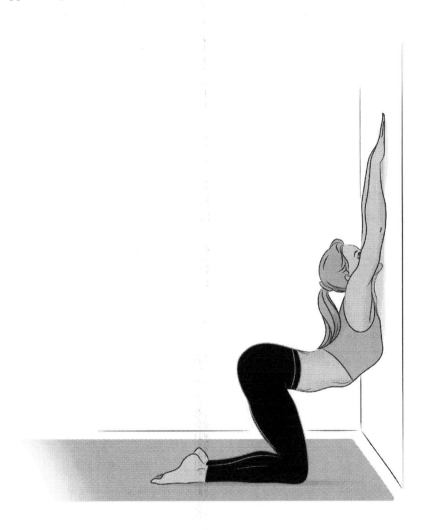

Puppy Dog Wall Pose Instructions

Starting Position

Begin by kneeling down about an arm's length away from a wall. Extend your arms in front of you and place your palms flat against the wall.

Pose 1

Begin to raise your hip and extend arms upward. Your head should naturally look upward and even feel a bit backward. This is similar to the feeling of the movement in exercise #1, the cow pose.

Pose 2

Deepen the stretch by gently pressing your palms into the wall and sinking your chest into it. Feel the stretch in your entire spine, neck, and abs.

Release

To release, simply sit your hips down onto your legs and relax your hands. Essentially, you are returning to the Lightning Pose (Exercise 10).

Tips:

- Remember, always move into and out of the pose gently and never force your body into a position that feels painful.

33 | Legs Up The Wall Pose

Using gravity, this pose re-aligns your hips and feels very relaxing.

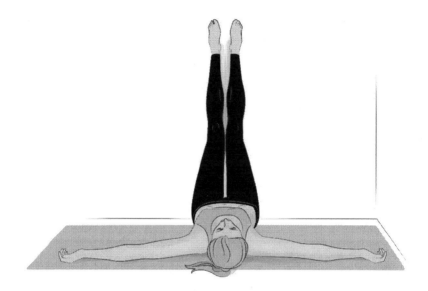

Legs Up The Wall Pose Instructions

Starting Position

Position your mat perpendicular to a wall to ensure a comfortable base for your back.

Sit sideways against the wall with 1 hip touching it.

Pose 1

Swing your legs up onto the wall as you lie back onto the mat. Adjust so your buttocks are close to or touching the wall, legs straight up.

Pose 2

Place arms at your sides, palms facing up.

Variations

A variation of this is to lay the arms sideways like a cross (pictured) or completely relaxed extended above your head on the mat.

Relax and breathe deeply, holding the pose for 30 seconds. Sometimes I stay here for up to a minute.

Release

To exit, bend knees, roll to one side, and gently push up to a seated position.

Tips:

- You can use a pillow or folded blanket under the lower back or hips for added support if needed.
- This pose with the hands fully extended like a cross is also found in the Egoscue Method, which re-aligns the hips and legs.

34 | Straddle Pose

This movement allows us to stretch both legs wide apart safely using gravity.

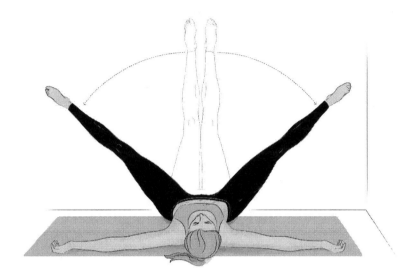

Straddle Pose Instructions

Starting Position

Position your mat perpendicular to a wall.

Sit sideways against the wall, with 1 hip touching it.

Swing your legs up onto the wall as you lie back onto the mat. Adjust so your buttocks are close to or touching the wall.

Pose 1

Extend legs straight up the wall.

Pose 2

Slowly open your legs into a "V" shape, letting gravity pull them down towards the floor. Go as far as you can comfortably.

Pose 3

Rest arms straight down each side. Relax and breathe deeply, holding the pose for as long as comfortable. I usually hold this for up to a minute because it feels so good.

To exit, gently use your hands to assist bringing legs back together, then bend knees and roll to one side.

Tips:

- If you can't extend your legs fully straight, don't worry. It's ok to bend them a little and to stretch only as far as you comfortably can.

35 | Wall Shoulder Stand

Using the wall for support, we're making the shoulder stand more accessible as an aligning and strengthening movement.

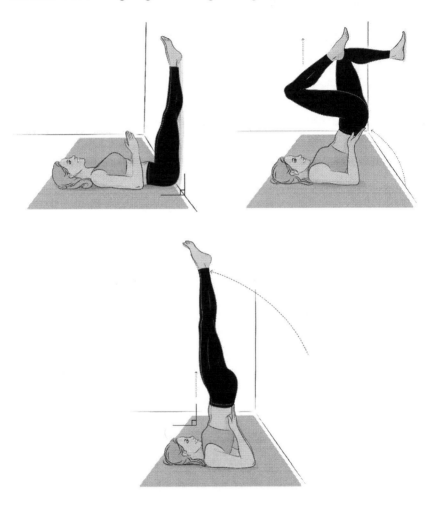

Wall Shoulder Stand Instructions

Starting Position

Position mat perpendicular to a wall. Lay down with feet facing it.

Wall "Just in case I fall" version:

Pose 1: Swing your feet upward in the air as you bring your hands to your back to stabilize your legs.

Pose 2: Press your hands into your waist and extend both legs straight up as far as you can without losing stability. Hold position for 20-30 seconds. Breathe deeply and mindfully.

Wall Assist Version:

Bring your legs up onto the wall as you lie back onto the mat. Adjust so your buttocks are close to or touching the wall.

Pose 1

Press your hands into your waist and walk both legs straight up the wall as far as you can without losing stability.

Pose 2

See if you can move your legs away from the wall while maintaining balance. See if you can hold position for 20-30 seconds. Breathe.

To exit, bend knees, slowly lower your spine down, and roll to one side.

Tips:

- The wall can act as a safety net if you lose balance. Just fall towards the wall and let the feet catch any potential falls. This allows you to feel comfortable extending as far as you can without a spotter.
- If you fall towards your head, ensure there's enough mat surface area to catch you or provide a soft landing.

36 | Wall Half Happy Baby Pose

This exercise stretches the hips, thighs, and groin. When practiced against a wall, it becomes an accessible variation for many individuals, offering support and allowing for a more controlled stretch.

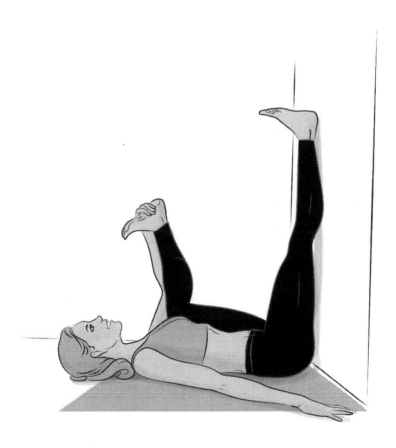

Wall Half Happy Baby Pose Instructions

Starting Position

Lay on your back close to a wall with your legs extended up it.

Easy Way: One way I do this is to scoot my buttocks close to the wall sitting sideways with the wall to my right, then turning clockwise to the right automatically raises both my legs against and close to the wall.

Pose 1

With your extended legs straight up the wall...now bend 1 knee (e.g., left knee) towards your chest.

Pose 2

Hold the outer edge of the foot (e.g., left foot) of the bent leg. Gently press the knee towards the floor beside your torso.

Relax and breathe, holding for a few seconds (I usually take 5 deep breaths here).

Switch and repeat with the other leg.

Tips:

- Keep your back flat on the floor.
- You can use a strap or belt around the foot if you can't comfortably reach it with your hand. Or, when starting out, you can just grab further up your ankles or calves.

37 | Half Plough Pose

This is a a great movement using the wall as support that stretches your lower back and legs.

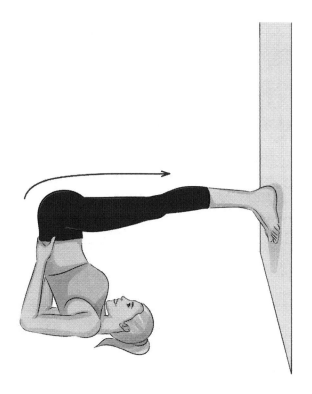

Half Plough Pose Instructions

Starting Position

Lay down with legs facing away from the wall and your head a few inches away.

Pose 1

Slowly kick your legs upward and backward until you reach the wall.

Pose 2

Ensure your legs are parallel to the floor and toes pointing downward.

You can lay your arms sideways on the floor or use them for stabilization by placing them to the sides of your core.

Breathe deeply and hold for a few seconds. I usually take 5 breaths here.

To exit, bend your legs and slowly roll to the side or swing your legs back into laying on the ground neutral.

Tips:

- Always be gentle with your spine and neck during this pose. If you feel any discomfort, come out of the pose.

38 | Standing Side Bend Pose

A simple yet effective exercise giving your sides an amazing stretch.

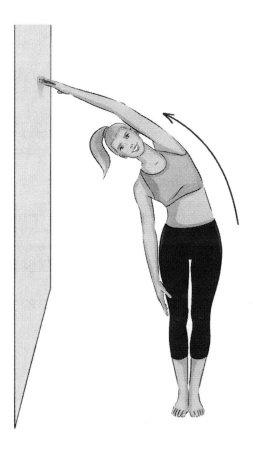

Standing Side Bend Pose Instructions

Starting Position

Stand sideways approximately an arm's length from a wall. Plant your feet firmly and closely together.

Pose 1

Extend the arm further from the wall overhead and place that hand on the wall for support. Take a deep breath in, and as you exhale, gently bend your torso for a deep stretch.

Pose 2

At the same time... the opposite arm can be extended alongside and down your body for another stretch. Hold for a few breaths, feeling the stretch along your sides.

Reverse Sides

Turn around and repeat on the opposite side for as many times as you like. I perform 3 stretches each side for about 15 seconds each.

Tips:

- Ensure you're bending from the waist, not the hips.
- Keep both feet grounded and maintain a soft bend in your knees to avoid locking them.
- Adjust distance from the wall as needed for comfort.

39 | Garland Pose With Wall

A deep squat that uses the wall for support while giving you a deep
stretch of the lower body.

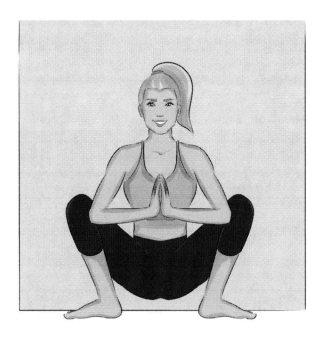

Garland Pose With Wall Instructions

Starting Position

Stand with your back to a wall, feet wider than hip-width apart. Turn your toes out slightly.

Pose 1

Begin to squat down, keeping your heels on the ground if possible. If heels lift, you can place a folded mat or blanket under them for support.

Allow your thighs to be wider than your torso, pressing your elbows against the inner knees.

Pose 2

Join your palms together in front of your heart. You can press your hips and even lower back gently against the wall for alignment and support.

Breathe deeply and hold for up to 30 seconds.

To release, press onto your feet and return to a standing position.

Tips:

- The wall provides support and helps in maintaining balance.
- Use your arms to push your legs even further out.
- As you get better, you can move away from using the wall. It's a beautiful movement either way.

40 | Standing Backbend Pose

A great way to open the font of the body for release. Be careful to only go as far as comfortable.

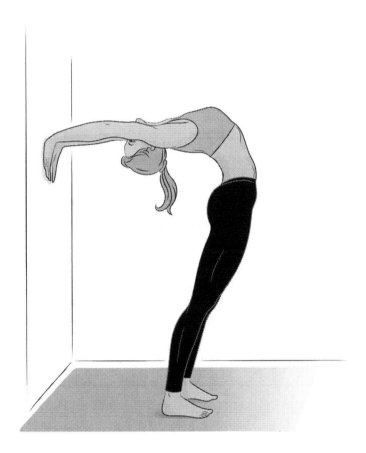

Standing Backbend Pose Instructions

Starting Position

Stand facing about a foot or two away from a wall, depending on your flexibility. Your feet should be comfortably apart.

Pose 1

Lean back and place your hands behind you on the wall, fingers pointing down.

Pose 2

Press into your feet, engaging your thighs and core. Begin to lift your chest upwards and arch your back. Allow the head to drop gently backward if comfortable.

Pose 3

Push against the wall with your hands for support and breathe deeply, holding the pose for up to 30 seconds.

To exit, engage your core and slowly lift the torso, returning to a neutral standing position.

Tips:

- You can keep a slight bend in the knees to avoid hyperextension.
- Always move within your comfort range to avoid straining the back and neck.

41 | Forward Fold Against Wall

This wall variation of the classic forward bend provides both muscle support and feedback, ensuring better spinal alignment.

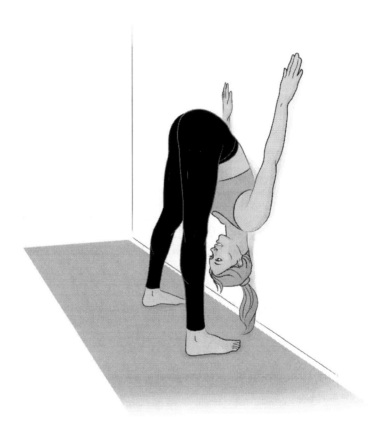

Forward Fold Against Wall Instructions

Starting Position

Stand a few feet away from a wall, facing it.

Keep feet hip-width apart and parallel to each other.

Pose 1

Lean forward and move your head down until your hands or upper body come in contact with the wall.

Pose 2

Press hips back to increase the stretch in the hamstrings and lower back.

Breathe deeply, holding for up to 30 seconds.

To exit, press into your feet and lift the torso, returning to standing.

Tips:

- Adjust the distance from the wall based on flexibility and comfort.
- Be careful not to hit your head on the wall the first few times. Go gently. You can also touch your head to the wall, then slowly slide down.

42 | Wall Butterfly Pose

The force of gravity, combined with the support of the wall, provides a gentle and effective stretch for your adductors and hamstrings.

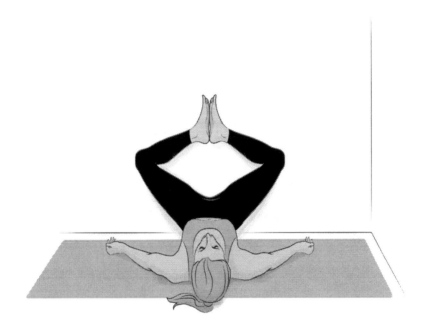

Wall Butterfly Pose Instructions

Starting Position

Sit on the floor with your buttocks positioned sideways to it. Lean to either side, which will automatically raise both legs against the wall.

Pose 1

Allow your legs to gently open, with your heels sliding down the wall towards your pelvis and forming a triangle shape with your legs.

Let both feet come together until they are pressing against each other.

Pose 2

Relax your arms to the floor on each side.

Variation

Bring your hands into a prayer pose.

Relax and breathe deeply, feeling a gentle inner thigh stretch.

To exit, roll to either side and gently extend your legs.

Tips:

- Adjust distance from the wall to change the intensity of the stretch.

43 | Wall Roll-Downs

This exercise is often used in physical therapy sessions to promote spinal mobility and awareness.

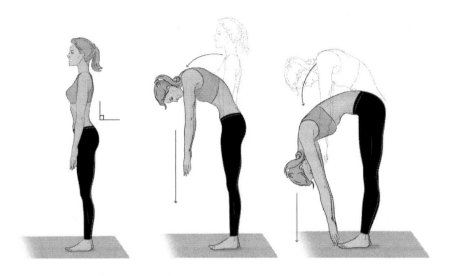

Wall Roll-Downs Instructions

Starting Position

Stand with your back against the wall for postural alignment, both arms comfortably lowered on each side. Your feet should be a few inches away from the wall. Butt can be touching the wall for another point of reference in your spinal alignment.

Pose 1

Tuck your chin to your chest.

Begin to roll down slowly by lowering your hands to the mat, allowing your back to round as you do.

If you're having trouble, bend the knees slightly as needed.

Pose 2

Pause for a breath at the bottom with the crown of your head pointing towards the floor.

Slowly roll back up to standing, re-stacking the spine, and lifting the head last.

Repeat 5 times.

Tips:

- This exercise promotes spinal flexibility and can be used to relieve tension in the back.
- Bend your knees if needed for comfort and to suit your flexibility.
- As you gain flexibility and can keep your legs and back straight then you'll no longer need to use the wall. I use it occasionally to check my alignment.
- If your flexibility improves, you can move your hands to hold in your elbows to create even more space to move further down.

Exercise Group Five

Pilates Routines With Strength Focus

The following exercises focus on increasing core strength.

Please warm up before attempting.

Remember that Pilates aspires for a balance of control and precision, but never at the expense of strength. We want balance between control, alignment, and flexibility because this works both the slow and fast-twitch muscles in your body.

If you're unsure about your ability to execute any of these exercises, please consult a certified Pilates teacher first.

44 | Wall Squats

This exercise uses the wall for support and ensures proper alignment for your lower body while strengthening the core.

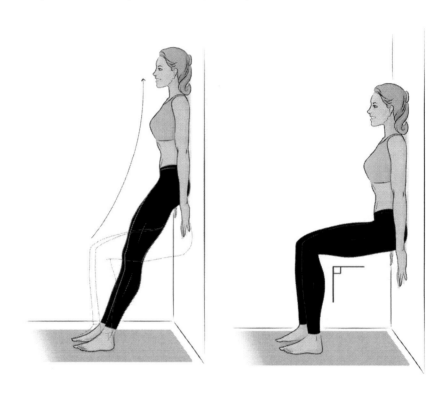

Wall Squats Instructions

Starting Position

Stand with your back against a wall, feet hip-width apart.

Pose 1

Slowly slide down the wall by bending your knees.

Lower until your thighs are parallel to the ground, or as far as comfortable.

Ensure your knees are directly above your ankles, forming a 90-degree angle.

Pose 2

Hold for 10 seconds (or longer based on endurance up to 60 seconds).

To exit: Slide back up to the starting position.

Tips:

- Engage your core throughout the exercise and breathe steadily.
- Adjust feet positioning if you feel any knee discomfort.
- The lower you go, the harder the hold. The higher, the easier.

45 | Wall Plank With Back Kick

A beautiful hip and leg strengthening exercise.

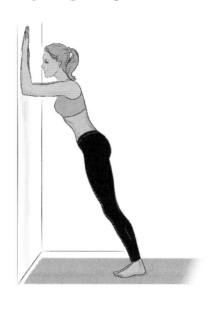

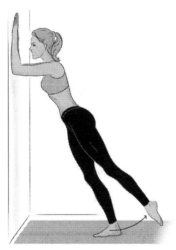

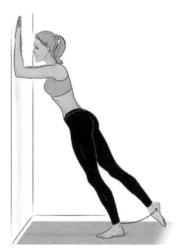

Wall Plank With Back Kick Instructions

Starting Position

Face the wall, standing a few feet away.

Pose 1

Extend your arms and lean your palms and forearms against the wall, shoulder-width apart.

Engage your core, ensuring a straight line from head to heels.

Pose 2

Move your left leg backward while maintaining the upper body plank position. Move back as high as you can. Return the leg back down.

Perform 3 times and each time see if you can go a little further.

Repeat 3 times with the right leg.

Return

To exit, place both feet on the ground and walk towards the wall.

Tips:

- Ensure you maintain a neutral spine and avoid sagging hips or arching the back.

46 | Wide-Legged Chair Pose

A variation pose that takes a wide stance with the toes pointing outward and thighs parallel to the ground.

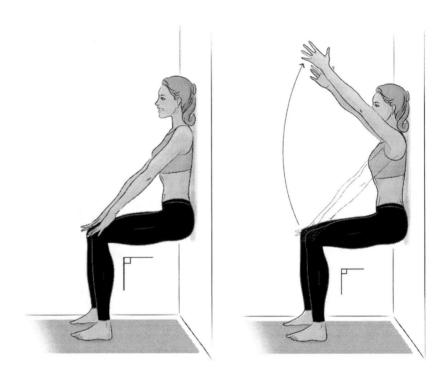

Wide-Legged Chair Pose Instructions

Starting Position

Stand with your back against a wall, feet wider than hip-width apart. For a more challenging hold, you can turn your toes slightly outwards.

Pose 1

Engage your core and bend your knees, sliding down the wall until your thighs are parallel to the ground (or as far as comfortable).

Ensure knees align with ankles and don't extend past your toes.

Pose 2

Extend arms out in front and raise them up into the sky.

You can press your buttocks against the wall for stability.

Hold the pose, breathing deeply. I usually stay here for up to 10 seconds.

To exit, press through your feet and slide back up to standing.

Tips:

- Ensure even weight distribution between both feet.
- The wall provides support and helps in maintaining alignment.
- Adjust the depth of the squat and hold time while squatting based on comfort.

47 | Wall Pike

An exercise with focus on the shoulders, core, and upper body. If you are unsure, please consult with a Pilates instructor. A spotter may help if you're new.

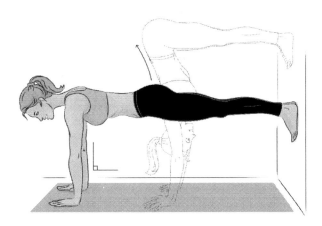

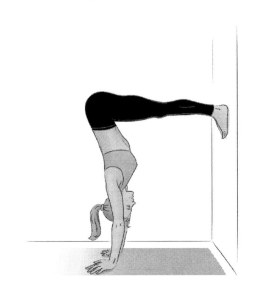

Wall Pike Instructions

Starting Position

Start in a plank position with your feet near the wall.

Pose 1

Walk your feet up the wall as you align your hands under your shoulders.

Pose 2

Now press palms firmly into the floor, spreading fingers wide.

Engage your core and move your hands backward and hips upward until your hips are directly on top of your shoulders and head.

Keep your head neutral between your arms, gazing towards your feet.

Hold the pose, breathing evenly. I usually stay here for 10-15 seconds.

To exit, carefully walk your feet down the wall to return to plank and stand up.

Tips:

- If you lose balance, I prefer to fall onto the side of the wall. This way you can regain your footing against the wall and try again.
- Don't feel the need to go beyond your means. Just move as far as you can. Some students just enjoy walking their feet up the wall and holding it there. As you gain strength and control eventually you will be able to perform a full wall pike.

48 | Wall Triceps Dips

Instead of using dumbbells, we press against a wall to target the triceps and surrounding muscle groups.

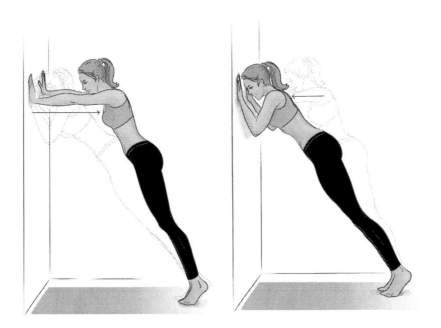

Wall Triceps Dips Instructions

Starting Position

Stand facing a wall, a few feet out. Place your hands on the wall, slightly wider than shoulder-width. Your body should be aligned like the Wall Plank exercise.

Pose 1

Keep elbows tucked in and lower down until your elbows press against the wall.

Pose 2

Push through your palms but isolate strength from your triceps to straighten your arms and lift your body back up.

Repeat this movement 10 times.

Tips:

- Adjust the difficulty by changing how far your feet are from the wall; farther away makes it more challenging.
- Ensure elbows don't flare out during the dip.
- While your body is at an angle to the wall, imagine your spine as a straight line from your neck down the tailbone, always aligned.

49 | Reverse Wall Plank

This exercise is particularly useful for individuals who might find the traditional reverse plank too challenging yet still want to strengthen their upper body.

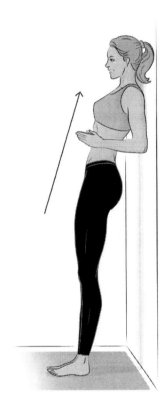

Reverse Wall Plank Instructions

Starting Position

Stand with you back facing the wall. Keep elbows tucked in and lean back down until your elbows are pressing against the wall.

Pose 1

Your body should form a straight line from your head to your heels with the elbow holding you up against the wall at a comfortable angle.

Engage your core and glutes, keeping your weight on your back heels.

Hold the position for a few breaths or as long as desired. I usually hold here for 15 seconds.

To exit, press into your toes and stand up straight

Tips:

- The wall provides a point of reference and support for maintaining alignment in this pose.
- Adjust elbow placement up or down for comfort if necessary.

50 | Wall Handstand

A wall assisted handstand works your core and upper body, as well as letting you practice control and concentration of balance for the whole body. Please use a spotter or consult a professional trainer if you cannot perform a handstand (yet).

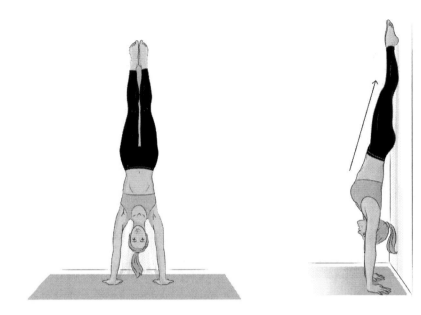

Wall Handstand Instructions

Starting Position

Find a sturdy wall with ample space in front and around. Stand facing the wall with 2 feet of space between your foot and the wall.

Pose 1

Place your hands on the floor about shoulder-width apart, about 1 foot away from the wall.

Pose 2

Kick up into a handstand, bringing both feet up against the wall.

Stack hips over shoulders and shoulders over wrists.

Keep fingers spread wide, pressing palms firmly into the ground.

Engage your core and legs, pointing toes towards the ceiling.

Hold the position, inhale, and exhale steadily for 3 breaths.

Return

To exit, carefully kick forward and descend 1 leg at a time, returning to starting position.

Tips:

- Begin with shorter hold durations and increase over time.
- Ensure your surroundings are safe and free from obstructions. A soft and large gym mat area may help with practicing handstands.
- If new to handstands, consider having a spotter or practice near a soft surface area.
- If you're unsure at all, please consult a certified trainer first.

51 | Wall Hundreds

A classic Pilates exercise performed for a count of 100. The Hundreds primarily target the core.

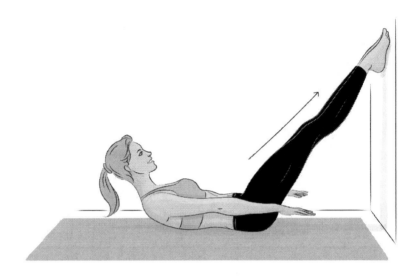

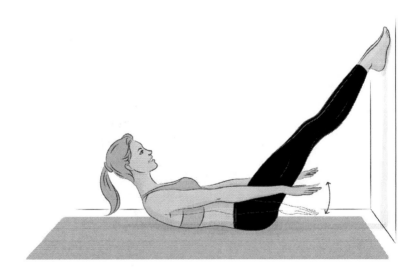

Wall Hundreds Instructions

Starting Position

Lie on your back, legs extended straight out at 45-degrees with feet pressing against the wall.

Pose 1

Lift head, neck, and shoulders off the mat, extending arms by your sides, palms facing down.

Pose 2

Pump your arms up and down in small, controlled movements. Inhale for 5 pumps, then exhale for 5.

See if you can do 100 pumps.

If you are new, experiment in increments of 20 (20, 40, 60, 80, 100).

After the pumps, relax head, neck, shoulders, and legs and melt into the floor.

Tips:

- Maintain core engagement and keep the lower back pressed into the mat.
- The name "hundreds" comes from the goal of 100 arm pumps. The breathing pattern and core engagement are essential components of the exercise.
- Modify by moving the feet lower or higher, or even flat on the ground or just slightly above the ground.
- As you improve, you can do this without the wall. Just raise your legs 2 inches off the floor, or even higher, up to 45-degrees into the air, and maintain balance with your core. At first you may need to bend your legs a bit until you develop enough strength to straighten them without the wall.

52 | Rotating Planks

AKA "Twisting Planks", this exercise adds to the traditional plank exercise with rotational movement and side planking, focusing on the upper body and core.

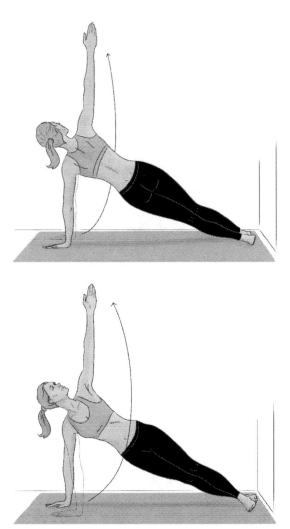

Rotating Planks Instructions

Starting Position

Begin in a standard plank position with arms straight, hands under shoulders, and body forming a straight line from head to heels. Heels are pressed against the wall for stability (optional).

Pose 1

Engage your core and shift your weight onto your left hand and rotate your body upward to the right, raising your right arm to the sky and coming into a side plank position.

Hold for a deep breath, then lower your right hand, returning to the standard plank position.

Pose 2

Repeat on the other side (left), rotating and placing weight onto your right hand and lifting your left arm into the sky. Hold for a deep breath, then return to plank position.

Continue alternating sides for 10 repetitions.

I perform 5 each side for a total of 10 reps.

Tips:

- You can modify this by dropping to your knees (easier).
- You can reduce difficulty by placing forearms on the mat instead of hands.
- You can remove your feet pressing against the wall for stability as you gain strength and balance.

53 | Leg Circles

This movement targets the muscles of the lower body.

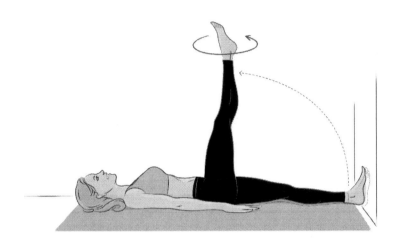

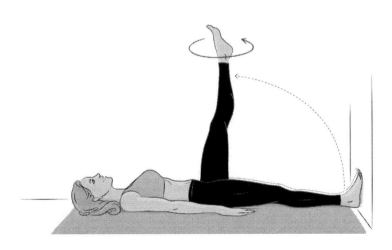

Leg Circles Instructions

Starting Position

Lie flat on your back on a mat. Arms should be resting by your sides with palms facing up. Ensure your neck and spine are aligned.

Wall Optional: Use the left foot to press into the wall for stability and to keep the left straight if it wants to lift up.

Pose 1

Lift Right Leg: Extend your right leg towards the ceiling, pointing your toes. Keep the left leg extended flat on the mat or slightly bent.

If you can't keep your right or left leg straight, don't worry, bend it a bit.

Circle Movement: Begin to circle your right leg clockwise towards the right side of the body. Carry out 5 controlled circles.

Repetitions: Switch to circling in the opposite direction (anti-clockwise).

Pose 2

Switch Legs: Lower your right leg and repeat the exercise with the other.

Wall Optional: Use the right foot to press into the wall for stability.

Modifications: If you have tight hamstrings, it's okay to have a slight bend in the knee.

If you want to challenge yourself further, lift the non-circling leg off the ground, holding it a few inches above the floor.

Tips:

- Always prioritize form over the size of the circle to avoid straining the back or hips.

54 | Wall Criss Cross

The "Criss Cross" is a classic movement that targets the abdominal muscles, especially the obliques.

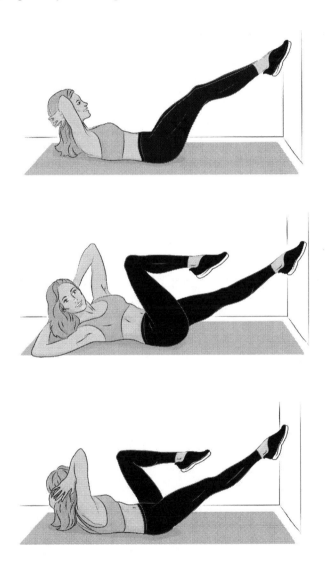

Wall Criss Cross Instructions

Starting Position

Starting Position: Lie on your back with hands behind your head and elbows wide. Lift your legs to a 45-degree angle, pressing your feet against the wall.

Engage Core: Press your lower back into the mat and engage your core muscles.

Pose 1

Lift head, neck, and shoulders off the mat. Rotate your left armpit towards your right knee as you bring the right knee in. Your left leg is stationary pressing against the wall.

Pose 2

Release back to neutral (first image).

Switch Sides

Now rotate to the opposite side, bringing your right armpit towards your left knee as the left knee comes in towards your head. Keep your right leg stationary pressing against the wall.

Repetitions: Continue alternating sides in a smooth, controlled manner for the desired reps. I perform 7 reps per side for a total of 14.

No Wall: As you get better you can move away from the wall supporting your non-moving leg. See if you can keep the non-moving leg straight. This really works out your core muscles.

Tips:

- Ensure your rotation comes from the ribcage and not just the elbows to maximize the exercise's benefits to your oblique muscles.
- Keep the movement controlled and avoid pulling on the neck.

55 | Wall Teaser

The "Teaser" is another iconic Pilates exercise known for its challenge and effectiveness. The wall variation requires less significant core strength, balance, and coordination. As you improve you can transition to using the floor only.

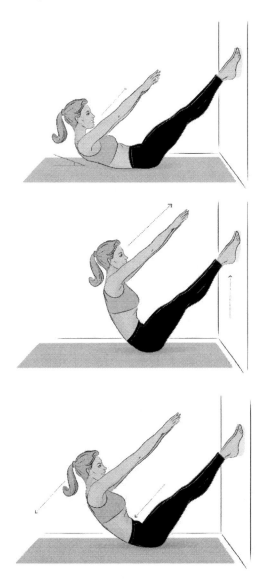

Wall Teaser Instructions

Starting Position

Lie on your back with legs extended at about a 45-degree angle using the wall as resistance. Rest arms on the floor with palms down.

Now lift your arms and head up towards the wall at a 45-degree angle.

Pose 1

Exhale as you lift your arms and head up further towards the wall.

Pose 2

Inhale as you bring your head, arms, back to starting position, still holding above the floor using your core. Keep your legs straight.

Repetitions: Repeat for the desired number of repetitions. I started out doing 10 controlled reps every morning, increasing by 5 each week. So, 10, 15, 20. Then I moved away from the wall and started again at 10.

Return: Slowly lower your upper body back down to the floor and walk your feet down from the wall.

No Wall: As you gain strength and control, see if you can do this without wall support for your legs. Try to keep your legs straight but it's ok with a little bend when starting out.

Tips:

- The Teaser is a challenging Pilates move that builds strength, balance, and control. Don't worry if you have to use the wall at first.
- The wall modification makes it easier to provide feedback when your movements are smooth and controlled because you don't need to think about the legs and can focus on the upper body movements.

56 | Wall Handstand Leg Extensions

A great way to build strength and stability in the shoulders, core, and legs. Please use a spotter if you're new to handstands and consider consulting an experienced Pilates instructor if you're unsure.

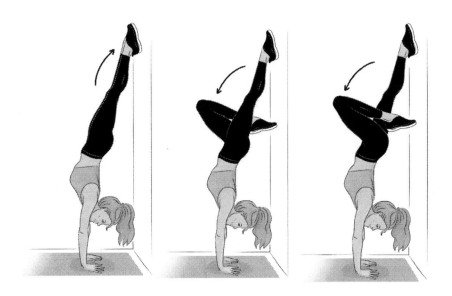

Wall Handstand Leg Extensions Instructions

Warning

Do not attempt this exercise without a spotter if you cannot do handstands yet! You can also try the easier variation explained in the tips section below.

Starting Position

Find a sturdy wall with ample space in front and around. Stand facing it with 2-3 feet of space between your foot and the wall.

Pose 1

Place your hands on the floor about shoulder-width apart, about 1-1.5 foot away from the wall. Kick up into a handstand so your heels are resting against the wall.

Pose 2

Keep your arms straight and directly below your shoulders. Engage your core and ensure your back is straight (avoid arching). Your body, from hands to feet, should form a straight line, perpendicular to the floor.

Pose 3

Slowly bend your left knees into a stretch. Your other leg should continue pointing up. Hold for 5 seconds and breathe.

Return & Repeat: Slowly raise the leg back up to meet the other leg against the wall. Now repeat the knee bend with the right leg.

Do this for 3 slow reps with each leg for a total of 6.

Exit: Carefully come out of the handstand by cartwheeling out to the side or pushing with your feet off the wall and cartwheeling 1 leg at a time into a standing position. Rest and shake out your wrists.

Tips:

- Keep your fingers spread wide and press through the base of your palms to distribute weight evenly.
- Breathe steadily; do not hold your breath.
- If new to this movement, consider having a spotter or practice on a soft surface first, like with a gym mat.
- **An Easier Variation:** Place both your forearms on top of your head. Hold your opposite elbows with your hands and use your elbows to balance yourself instead of your hands. Then kick your legs into the wall and just do the leg movements without the handstand. Use your elbows and head instead for balance.

Next Steps

"Pilates is not what you get, it is what you give to yourself[1]"

— *John Howard Steel*

Once you get into the habit of these movements, you won't want to stop. Use the 28-Day Challenge programs to stay motivated and on track.

After a while... doing Pilates to feel more flexible, stronger, toner and vibrant every day just becomes an addictive habit!

I know that some of you will want to continue onto more advanced exercises, so before we say goodbye, let me direct you to our exclusive Pelvic Floor Kegels exercise at wallpilates.org as taught by Tim Sawyer, a leading physical therapist who worked with Dr. Anderson and Dr. Wise at the Stanford University Medical Center[2]. When you enter your email to download this free bonus, you'll also be notified of new Pilates books and workout routines we'll release in the future. Just go to wallpilates.org and get all your 4 FREE bonuses.

You can also scan the following QR code to receive your free bonuses:

---

1. Steel, John Howard. Caged Lion: Joseph Pilates and His Legacy (p. 181). Last Leaf Press. Kindle Edition.
2. Authors of A Headache in the Pelvis: A New Understanding and Treatment for Chronic Pelvic Pain Syndromes.

Thank You

My name is Luna and it has been my pleasure to serve you.

You could have picked from dozens of other books but you took a chance and chose this one.

So, thank you for investing in yourself and making it to the end!

Before we say goodbye, one question: if you enjoyed this book, would you consider leaving a review? A review is the easiest and best way to support the work of independent authors like me. Your feedback will help me continue writing the types of books that will help you and others in the journey to good health:

Please Leave a review here:
> Wall Pilates Book 1

Pilates is a safe, effective, and beautiful movement technique that helps clients improve their lives. From recovering from chronic pain, to staying in shape as we age, to feeling stronger and healthier... it adds value no matter which stage of life you're living right now.

As you work on these exercises, by the fifth or sixth session, you will start to feel more aligned in your posture and feel like you're standing taller.

By the tenth session, you won't want to stop.

By the twentieth session it will become a habit.

This technique, invented by Joseph Pilates, literally gave me my life back after a car accident. I hope now, with the exercises in this book, you can enjoy all these benefits Pilates has to offer you from the comfort of your own home.

At the beginning of this book, I made a bold claim that "practicing Pilates will make you happier and healthier."

Do you feel happier? Healthier? I hope so, and for those of you who enjoy reading but have yet to start the exercises, I'd like to end with a quote you read at the start of this book from Joseph Pilates himself:

> *"In 10 sessions, you'll feel the difference. In 20, you'll see the difference. And in 30, you'll be on your way to having a whole new body."*[1]

— Joseph Pilates

If you haven't started yet, what are you waiting for? Try out these movements for yourself and feel the truth in your body.

To your happiness and health,
-Luna Light

P.S.

If you enjoyed the book, I would appreciate it so much if you took a few seconds to leave us your thoughts on Amazon so we can share the wonders of Pilates with more people. Thank you in advance for supporting independent writers like me.

P.S.S.

There are several people that deserve the credit. My partner, my family, my publishing contacts, and all of my friends who inspired me and helped me complete this book. I could not have done it without them, especially when I was recovering from chronic pain.

And thank you, the reader, for making it this far and for your support for independent authors like me.

---

1. Pilates, Joseph, H.; Miller, William, John. Return to Life Through Contrology.

Additional Resources

Use this URL from the National Pilates Certification Program to find a certified Pilates instructor:
https://nationalpilatescertificationprogram.org/NPCP/NPCP/Directory/CertifiedTeachersList.aspx

Joseph Pilate's original exercise book:
Return To Life Through Contrology

The personal life of Pilates from the perspective of one of his students and close friends, John Howard Steel:
Caged Lion: Joseph Pilates & His Legacy

The Philosophy and Principles of Pilates.
First published in 1934, this book includes Joseph Pilates' early Twentieth Century philosophies, principles, and theories about health and fitness:
Your Health: A Corrective System of Exercising That Revolutionizes the Entire Field of Physical Education

Citations

Cover Image Source: Free license from Freepik.com

Disclosures

Some of the links provided in this book are affiliate links, which help you jump to the exact URL of the resource you're looking for at no additional cost to you.

The Legal Stuff

Assumption of Risk: By reading/using this book, the User/Reader acknowledges that physical exercise involves inherent risks and hazards. By choosing to follow or participate in any exercise regimen, instruction, or advice detailed in the Book, the User expressly and voluntarily assumes all risks associated with such activities, recognizing that they may result in injury, illness, death, and/or damage to personal property.

Waiver: By reading this book/guide, The User hereby waives, releases, and forever discharges the author, publisher, and all related parties from any and all claims, liabilities, actions, suits, demands, costs, losses, damages, attorney's fees, and expenses, whether known or unknown, foreseen, or unforeseen, that arise out of or relate to the User's/Reader's use of or reliance on the Book/Workout Guide.

Made in the USA
Las Vegas, NV
29 March 2025

99a0010c-ca06-4c78-ac0f-1aa0230eae5eR01